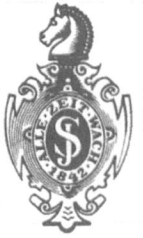

Springer-Verlag France S.A.R.L

D. Gossot, Ph. Kleinmann, J.F. Levi (Eds.)

Surgical thoracoscopy

with contributions by :
P. Baldeyrou, S. Barker, P.A. Belloni, J. Bourcereau, J. Byrne, N. Gharbi,
W.P. Hederman, P.D. Ridley, M. Torre, N. Trivedi, A. Wakabayashi, T.N. Walsh

With 121 Figures

Preface by D.J. Sugarbaker

Springer-Verlag France S.A.R.L

D. Gossot, MD
Department of Surgery
Saint-Louis Hospital
75010 Paris, France

Ph. Kleinmann, MD
Department of Thoracic Surgery
Clinique Bachaumont
75002 Paris, France

J.F. Levi, MD
Department of Thoracic Surgery
Marie-Lannelongue Hospital
92350 Le Plessis-Robinson, France

Cover picture : View of the mediastinum through the thoracoscope (Photograph : D. Gossot).

© Springer-Verlag France, 1992
Originally published by Springer-Verlag France in 1992
Softcover reprint of the hardcover 1st edition 1992

The use of registered names, trademarks, etc. in this publication does not imply, even in the absence of a specific statement, that such names are exempt from the relevant protective laws and regulations and therefore free for general use.
Product Liability : The publisher can give no guarantee for information about drug dosage and application there of contained in this book. In every individual case the respective user must check its accuracy by consulting other pharmaceutical litterature.

ISBN 978-2-8178-0896-3   ISBN 978-2-8178-0894-9 (eBook)
DOI 10.1007/978-2-8178-0894-9

2918/3917/543210. Printed on acid free paper.

Table of contents

Thoracoscopic treatment of pneumothorax (A-D)

Preface

Minimally invasive surgical techniques have made a significant impact in lowering morbidity and mortality and in changing the indications for operative surgery in the abdomen. Only recently have these minimally invasive techniques been applied to the diseases of the thorax. The standard posterior lateral thoracotomy infamous for its post-operative pain and attendant complications, is already being replaced in a large number of situations by minimally invasive thoracoscopic techniques.

This text by Gossot, Kleinmann and Levi provides basic information required for surgeons interested in approaching the most common diseases in the chest utilizing thoracoscopic techniques. The text is a well organized attempt to acquaint surgeons with basic thoracoscopic surgery. Basic instrumentation for thoracoscopic surgery is well outlined and discussed and will allow surgeons to become readily familiar with this rapidly changing field of surgical instrumentation.

Thoracoscopic surgery utilizes some basic principles of surgical technique and draws upon newer principles based on advanced instrumentation. These concepts are well covered in the section on basic techniques and thoracoscopic surgery by Dr. Gossot. This new disciplined way of thinking allows surgeons to begin to formulate surgical approaches to particular disease entities as required by this surgical approach.

Thoracoscopic anesthesia is different from traditional thoracic anesthesia. Vast differences in post-operative pain and discomfort attendant to the minimally invasive procedure allow for modifications in anesthetic technique. The basics of this endeavor are well covered in this section.

The basic techniques of thoracoscopic surgery were developed in various diagnostic maneuvers. It was this initial diagnostic application of thoracoscopy which allowed these techniques to be developed and further therapeutic applications to be forwarded. This text nicely illustrates current diagnostic techniques and their application.

In addition, the most commonly applied therapeutic procedures in the pleura, lung and esophagus are well covered as are their indications and potential complications.

Drs. Gossot, Kleinmann and Levi are to be congratulated for their well organized effort to present fundamental aspects of thoracoscopic surgery utilizing text presented by leaders in this field.

It appears clear that the applications for thoracoscopic surgery are to be limited only by the imagination of the surgeons applying these techniques to a wide variety of disease entities. We stand at an exciting vista with a potential new « century of the surgeon » as surgeons once again develop new operative techniques for the treatment of surgical disease.

David J. Sugarbaker, M.D.
Chief, Division of Thoracic Surgery
Brigham & Women's Hospital
Harvard Medical School
Boston, MA 02115, USA

Acknowledgements

We wish to thank all the authors who collaborated with us on this book and who gave of their experience. Special thanks to Akio Wakabayashi for his generous contribution.

We are very grateful to Olympus for their support and their technical assistance. We especially thank Mrs C. Boras, Mr J.F. Deniau, Mr M. Deretz, Mrs M. Löffler, Dr T. Lüdtke, Mr A. Shiga, Mr A. Taguchi, Dr S. Trispel and Mr R. Zentner for their help in the development of thoracoscopic instrumentation.

List of authors

P. Baldeyrou, MD
Department of Pneumology, Porte de Choisy Hospital, 75013 Paris, France

S.J. Barker, MD
Department of Anesthesiology, University of California, Irvine, California 92717, U.S.A.

P.A. Belloni, MD
Department of Thoracic Surgery, A.De Gasperis, Niguarda Hospital, Milano 20131, Italy

J. Bourcereau, MD
Department of Thoracic and Vascular Surgery, Marie-Lannelongue Hospital, 92350 Le Plessis Robinson, France

J. Byrne, FRCSI
Department of Surgery, University College Hospital, Galway, Ireland

N. Gharbi, MD
Department of Thoracic and Vascular Surgery, Marie-Lannelongue Hospital, 92350 Le Plessis Robinson, France

D. Gossot, MD
Department of Surgery, Saint-Louis Hospital, 75010 Paris, France

W.P. Hederman, MCh, FRCSI
Department of Surgery, Mater Misericordiae Hospital, Dublin 1, Ireland

Ph. Kleinmann, MD
Department of Thoracic Surgery, Clinique Bachaumont, 75002 Paris, France
American Hospital of Paris, 92202 Neuilly-sur-Seine, France

J.F. Levi, MD
Department of Thoracic Surgery, Marie-Lannelongue Hospital, 92350 Le Plessis Robinson, France
Department of Thoracic Surgery, Clinique Bachaumont, 75002 Paris, France

P.D. Ridley, BA, MBBS, FRCS, MA, MD
Department of Cardiothoracic Surgery, Bristol Royal Infirmary, Bristol, England

M. Torre, MD
Department of Thoracic Surgery, A. De Gasperis, Niguarda Hospital, Milano 20131, Italy

N.S. Trivedi, MD
Department of Anesthesiology, University of California, Irvine, California 92717, U.S.A.

A. Wakabayashi, MD, FACS, Dr. Med. Sci.
Department of Surgery, University of California, College of Medicine, Irvine, California 92717, U.S.A.

T.N. Walsh, MCh, FRCSI
Department of Clinical Surgery, St. James's Hospital, Dublin 8, Ireland

Introduction

D. Gossot

Thoracoscopy is both a very old and a very new surgical technique. It was first used around 1910 after Jacoboeus, using cystoscopic instruments, had demonstrated that this technique was useful for the lysis of pleural adhesions and for pneumothorax therapy for pulmonary tuberculosis [6]. The technique was subsequently developed mainly because thoracic surgery did not then exist as such [8, 9]. With the advent of modern thoracic surgery and sophisticated anesthetic techniques, thoracic surgeons neglected thoracoscopy and considered it a minor technique, because it was thought that nothing could offer all the options that would be provided by a wide posterolateral thoracotomy. Starting from the 1960's, all minor and major thoracic operations were performed with a minimal and reasonably low mortality rate. However, both high post-operative morbidity rate [5, 7] and painful post-operative course were considered the price one had to pay for chest surgery.

Only pneumologists continued to consider thoracoscopy as a valuable diagnostic technique and some developed useful procedures for pleural and lung biopsies, using specific instrumentation [1, 2, 4, 10]. Some therapeutic techniques such as pleurodesis were also included in their field of interest [11]. However, the development of these techniques was limited by the need to avoid complications which could requiring thoracotomy. Thoracoscopy and open chest surgery have thus followed separate but parallel routes for many years. However their paths have recently crossed with the marked evolution of endoscopic surgery. An increasing number of thoracic surgeons are now convinced that minimal invasive surgery is one of the ways to reduce operative trauma without compromising exposure of the operative field [3, 12]. The proportion of all thoracic procedures that can be performed by thoracoscopy has not yet been established. Meanwhile, ideas, techniques and equipment are advancing so fast that it already seems obsolete to open the chest to treat a recurrent spontaneous pneumothorax or perform a lung biopsy [12]. However, numerous fields are still unexplored and many avenues of research are still open.

This book is for surgeons. For this reason, many basic aspects of anatomy or technique which are familiar to them have been omitted. On the other hand, some major procedures which have been endoscopically performed sporadically, but which are still only case-reports have not been included. As far to the techniques on which general agreement has not yet been reached, such as the endoscopic treatment of pneumothorax, we have preferred to describe the various procedures currently performed and to let the reader make up his own mind. Some readers may be surprised to encounter chapters on diagnostic thoracoscopy. We believe that the theoretic barriers between medical and operative thoracoscopy are becoming increasingly blurred. One of the benefits of rediscovering thoracoscopy is the rediscovery of the forgotten and exciting field of diagnostic endoscopy.

References

1. Brandt HJ (1977) Endoskopie und Biopsie in der Diagnostik pneumologischer Krankheiten. Prax Pneumol 31 : 384-401
2. Boutin C, Viallat JR, Cargnino P, Rey F (1982) Thoracoscopic lung biopsy. Experimental and clinical preliminary study. Chest 82 : 44-48
3. Cushieri A (1991) Minimal Access Surgery and the future of interventional laparoscopy. Am J Surg 161 : 404-407

4. Guérin JC, Champel F, Biron E, Kalb JC (1985) Talcage pleural par thoracoscopie dans le traitement du pneumothorax. Etude d'une série de 109 cas traités en 3 ans. Rev Mal Respir 2 : 25-29

5. Hallfeldt KKJ, Knoeffel WTK, Thetter O, Deubler E, Schweiberer L (1990) Respiratory function after thoracic operations. Ann Thorac Surg 50 : 684-685

6. Jacobaeus HC (1910) Über die Möglichkeit, die Zystoskopie bei Untersuchung seröser Höhlungen anzuwenden. Münch Med Wochenschr 40 : 2090-2092

7. Sabanathan S, Eng J, Mearns AJ (1990) Alterations in respiratory mechanics following thoracotomy. J R Coll Surg Edinb 35 : 144-150

8. Sattler A (1937) Zur Behandlung des Spontanpneumothorax mit besonderer Berücksichtigung der Thorakoskopie. Beitr Klin Tuberk 89 : 395-408

9. Sergent E, Kourilsky R (1939) Contribution à l'étude de l'endothéliome pleural. Images radiologiques et pleuroscopiques. Presse Méd 14 : 257-259

10. Swierenga J, Wagenaar JP, Bergstein PG (1974) The value of thoracoscopy in the diagnosis and treatment of diseases affecting the pleura and lung. Pneumologie 151 : 11-18

11. Thermann M, Loddenkemper R, Schröder D (1985) Thoracoscopy : a forgotten endoscopic procedure ? Endoscopy 17 : 203-204

12. Wakabayashi A (1991) Expanded application of diagnostic and therapeutic thoracoscopy. J Thorac Cardiovasc Surg 102 : 721-723

Instrumentation for thoracoscopic surgery

D. Gossot

Thoracoscopic equipment is similar to laparoscopic equipment. The optical systems and some of the instrumentation are similar. However, some of the thoracoscopic instruments and equipment are specialised.

1. Optical system

1.1. Endoscopes

The use of an intercostally introduced mediastinoscope has been proposed [9], but its manipulation is not as convenient as the manipulation of modern telescopes.

In diagnostic thoracoscopy, the use of 7 mm-telescopes is possible [2, 14]. But in operative thoracoscopy accurate dissection requires a large field of view and a large depth of field. These needs require a high degree of brightness and a high resolution which can only be obteined with 10 mm optics. The rigid 10 mm laparoscope is one the most used [13, 16]. In children, a 5 mm instrument, or 4 mm in infants [15], is sufficient because of the small size of the chest and is easier to manipulate.

At least two telescopes are required: one with direct vision (0°) and one with an angulated view (30°). The latter has the advantage of reducing the dead angle, which is particularly troublesome when examining areas such as the lateral chest wall. There are also 45° telescopes, but they are more difficult to manipulate and are not used very often. Where indicated, as in laser dissection, it is useful to have an operating telescope with an integrated operating channel (Fig. 1). None of the rigid telescopes, whatever their direction of view, allows a complete examination of the chest and thus does not totally solve the problem of the dead angle. This problem is more troublesome than in laparoscopic surgery, because of the rigidity of the chest, which is why some authors have proposed using a flexible bronchoscope [4, 20, 21]. The disadvantage of the bronchoscope is its relatively poor brightness and resolution. The flexibility of the inserted portion also leads to manipulative problems because of the limited intercostal space. The solution is to use a superior optic having a rigid insert with a flexible tip. The development of such endoscopes is in progress. A 9 mm model is already commercially available (Fig. 2).

The rigid endoscope is connected to a camera and a cold light source.

1.2. Light source

The most commonly used cold light sources are xenon or halogen lamps. The advantages of the xenon light source are the natural light color – the halogen lamp is much more yellow – and the better conversion rate from electrical power into light. This leads to improved brightness compared to the halogen lamp even if the same power is used. For video documentation, a 300 W-xenon light source is recommended, such as the Olympus CLV-S or CLV-U20 (Fig. 3). Automatic control of the light intensity is necessary in order to avoid overexposure of the tissues in close-up views.

1.3. Camera

The CCD camera (charge-coupled-device) has a high resolution and high degree of sensitivity. Most

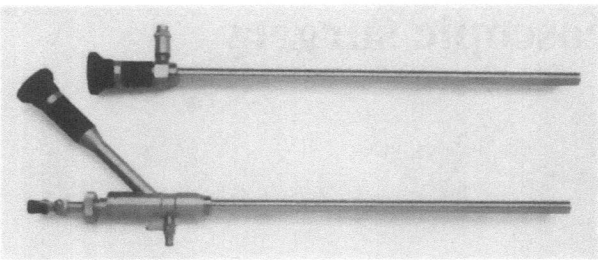

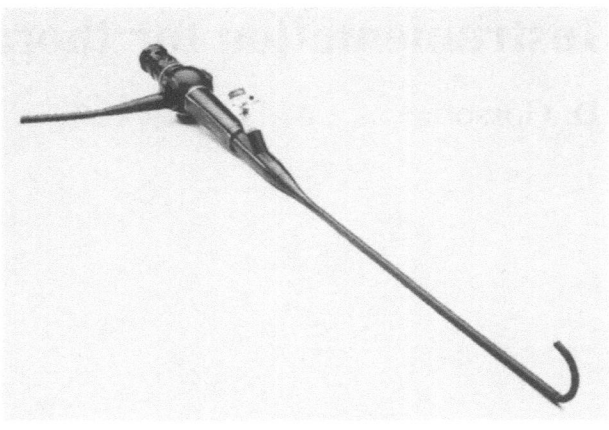

Fig. 1. 10 mm-0° telescopes (Olympus)

Fig. 2. Rigid 9 mm fiberoptic thoracoscope with flexible tip (Olympus)

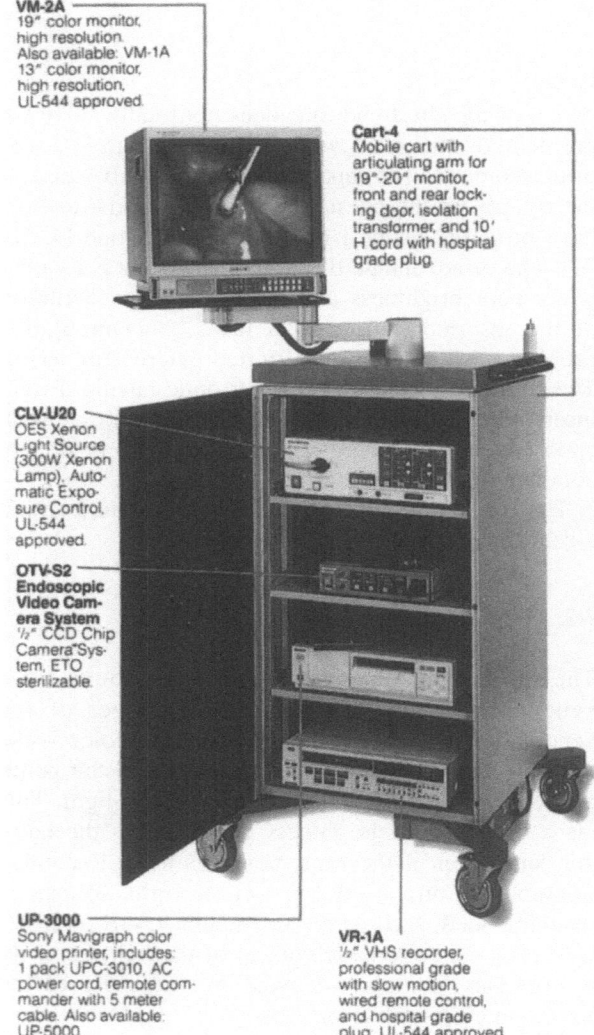

Fig. 3. Video-trolley with contents : high-resolution TV-Monitor (Sony), xenon-light Source (Olympus), OTV-S2 Olympus Camera, video-printer (Sony) and VHS recorder (Sony)

modern cameras have an automatic control for white balance and colors. The Olympus OTV-S2 camera system has a small size and weight which make it easy to manipulate (Fig. 3). The camera can be connected to the endoscope either through a direct connector (Fig. 4a) or through an adaptor (Fig. 4b). This latter mechanism is more convenient when several telescopes are used, but has the disadvantage of being more sensitive to fogging. The camera is connected to a high-resolution TV monitor.

For maximal comfort it is advisable to use two large screen monitors, one on each side of the operating table.

2. Irrigation-suction system

Introduction of the irrigation fluid by gravity may be sufficient in some minor diagnostic procedures. However, in most cases it is safer to use a device using irrigation under pressure, such as the Endo-Rinse (Figs. 5 and 6) which breaks up clots and permits rapid clearing of the operative field. In some cases, the Surgimat with its pressure control for irrigation is also useful for hydrodissection.

3. Electrocautery

The bipolar coagulation which is recommended by some laparoscopic surgeons [18] is rarely helpful in thoracoscopic surgery. Monopolar cautery is used more often and most of the instruments can be connected to the cautery. At the present time, only foot-control of the cautery is available and this may give rise to severe accidental burns. The monopolar cautery is as effective as the laser [6, 8, 10, 17] for

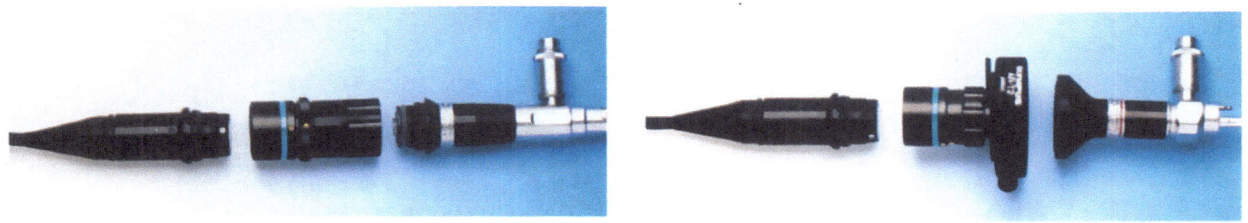

a   b

Fig. 4a, b. Telescope-camera adapters with **a** direct coupling and **b** clamped connection (Olympus)

most pleural and mediastinal dissections. However, it is both difficult and hazardous to apply on lung parenchyma.

4. Lasers

For the surgeon the acronym LASER (Light Amplification by Stimulated Emission of Radiation) means an instrument with which he can perform both cutting and coagulation at the same time. Moreover, the laser can be used for a wide field of other medical applications in diagnostics and therapeutics. The light a laser emits has many advantages such as high intensity, small beam divergence and specific wavelengths. Most lasers used in medicine only emit one wavelength and this is important because the effect on the tissue is mainly a function of the amount of energy transferred to a limited area. As in HF techniques it is possible to perform cutting and coagulation by varying the wavelength, the power, the tip of the fiber used and the distance from the tissue. The final effect is influenced not only by the laser characteristics but also by the physical properties of the tissue, such as the absorption index which depends strongly on the wavelength and the chemical composition of the tissue. Several lasers for general surgery are available: carbon dioxide (CO_2), neodynium-YAG (Nd-YAG), argon-ion and frequency-doubled Nd-YAG lasers (short KTP lasers).

- The CO_2 laser emits an invisible infrared beam (10.6 μm). The laser medium itself is made up of a mixture of carbon dioxide, nitrogen and helium. For its excitation a radio frequency or an electric discharge is used. Its energy is well absorbed by the cellular water as by the hemoglobin and the light is less scattered. This result in a superficial injury of the tissue and in a "what you see is what you get" effect. It is the ideal laser for vaporisation, e.g in bleb excision [3]. However, this superficial effect makes it difficult to use for dissection or achieving hemostasis [6, 8, 10].

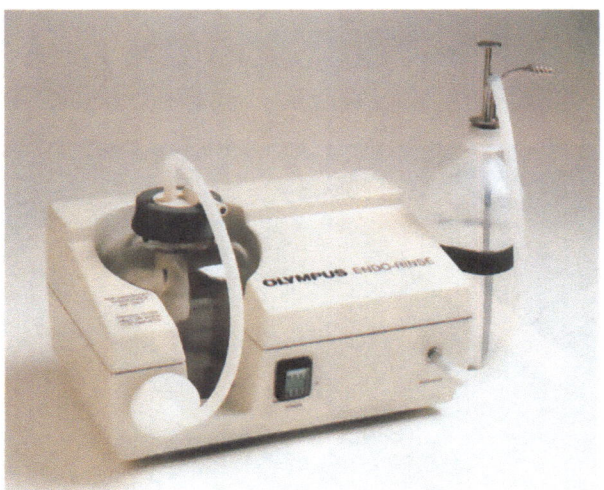

5

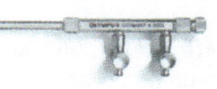

6

Fig. 5. Irrigation pump (Olympus)

Fig. 6. Suction-irrigation tube (Olympus)

- The Nd-YAG laser works in the invisible near infrared with a wavelength of 1.064 μm. Normally, the neodynium-doped yttrium aluminium garnet crystal is excited for laser activity by a flash lamp. Unlike the CO_2 laser, it can be passed through flexible quartz fibers making it very suitable as an endoscopic tool. Its energy can be transmitted through water and is intensely absorbed in tissue protein the energy being scattered throughout the tissue. These effects result in a deep penetration of energy, giving rise to greater damage below the surface than on the surface itself. This often leads to underestimation of the

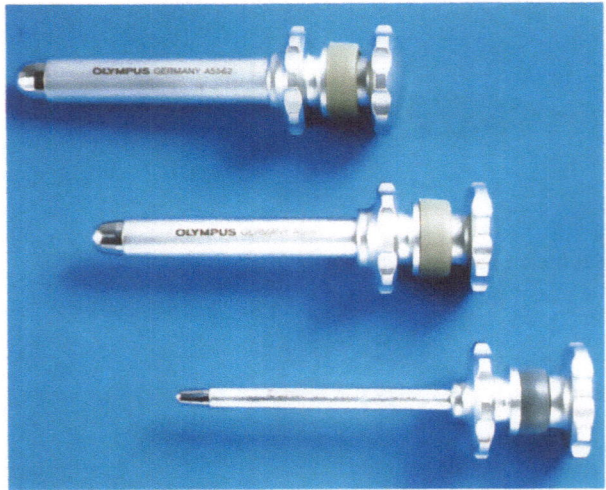

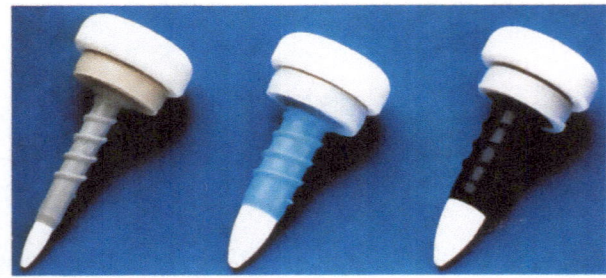

7

8

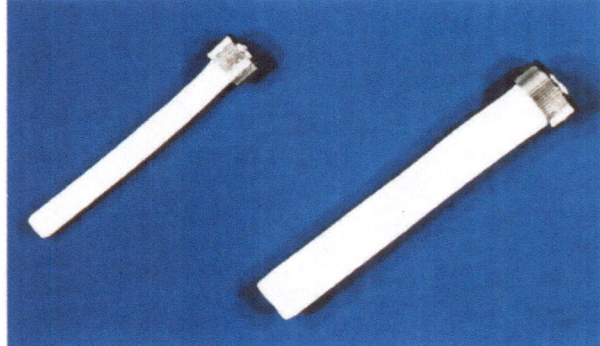

9

Fig. 7. Reusable thoracoscopic trocar tubes (Olympus)

Fig. 8. Disposable thoracoscopic trocar tubes (USSC)

Fig. 9. Flexible thoracoscopic trocar tubes for insertion of curved instruments (Olympus)

effect [10], but the recent availability of sapphire tips which can be attached to the quartz fibers means that it can be used in a contact mode thus making effect control much safer [17, 23]. By using different probes of various shapes, it is possible to get scalpel effects as well as a coagulation or vaporisation effect.

- The argon-ion or short argon laser emits light in the visible blue/green range between 0.488 μm and 0.514 μm. The laser medium argon gas is excited by an electrical discharge and is primarily operated in a continuous mode. Because the wavelength is visible, no expensive quartz fibers are needed for transmitting the beam and it passes through water without further absorption. It can therefore be applied directly through an operative telescope or with a fiber. If only a cutting effect is to be obtained, the fiber is better used in contact with the tissue than in a noncontact mode. Argon laser light can penetrate deeply into tissues up to 6 mm.

- The KTP laser is a frequency-doubled Nd.YAG laser. KTP crystal (potassium titanyl phosphate) converts the 1.064 μm radiation of the Nd-YAG laser into visible radiation at 532 μm. Wavelength and power output are very similar to the argon laser

which results in similar characteristics. The good absorption by hemoglobin makes it well suited for coagulation.

Because laser technology is rather expensive at the moment and because it is hard to imagine having all the various types of lasers in the operating room, the Nd.YAG laser used in a contact mode with different probes seems to be most suitable [1, 5, 11, 12, 22]. However, the use of lasers in thoracoscopic surgery is mainly limited to the treatment of some blebs and bullae. So, their acquisition and choice have to be considered thoroughly .

5. Instrumentation

Some thoracoscopic instruments are identical to those used for surgical laparoscopy, but for most thoracoscopic procedures specific instrumentation is required. It is easier and more convenient to use only 5 and 10 mm devices, in order to reduce the number of maneuvers and to avoid equipment incompatibility.

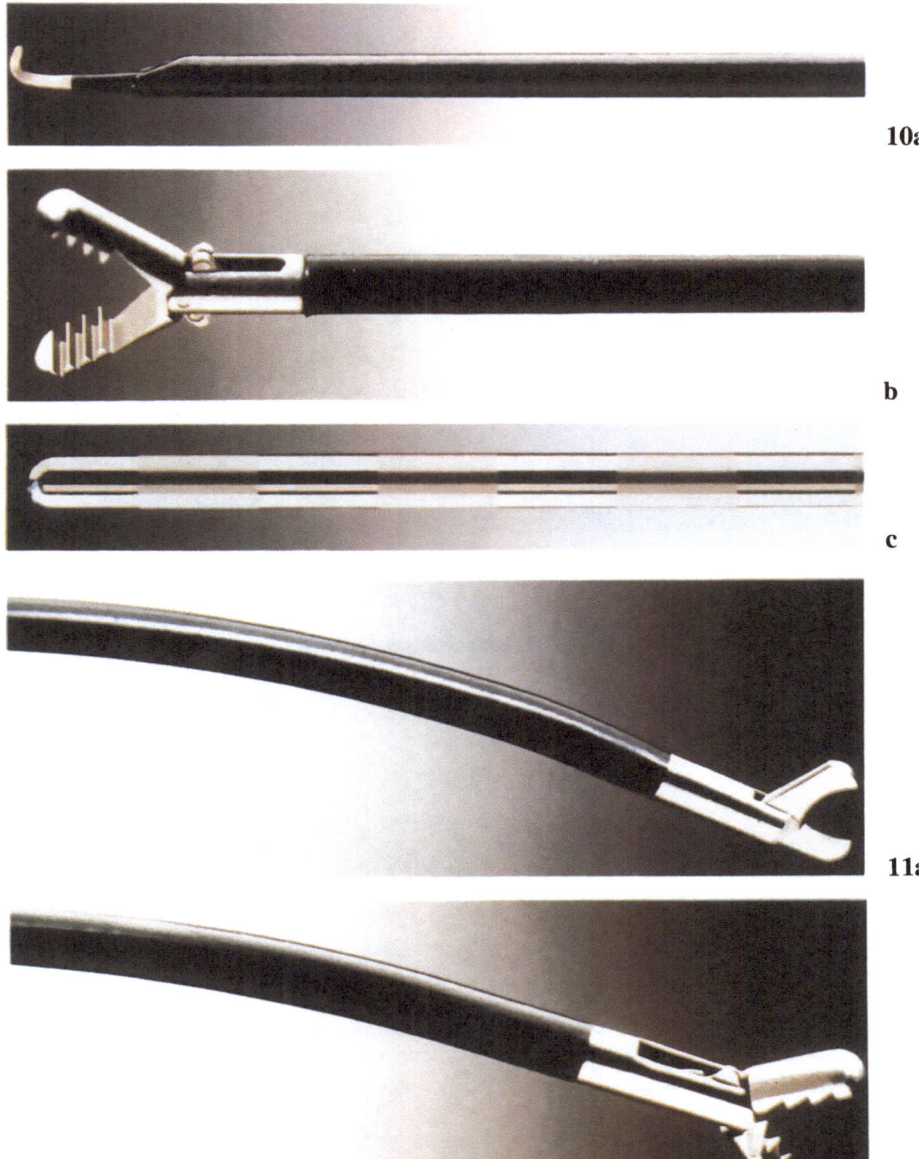

Fig. 10a-c. Straight instruments (Olympus). **a** Coagulating hook, **b** biopsy forceps, **c** palpation probe

Fig. 11a, b. Curved instruments (Olympus): **a** Hook scissors, **b** biopsy forceps

5.1. Trocars

Laparoscopic trocar tubes are unsuitable for thoracoscopy. Their sharp trocar point may cause lung injuries and they are too long, thus impeding vision when they enter the operating field. Their air-tight piston valve is not only unnecessary but awkward. Short trocars with a blunt tip and trocar tubes without a valve mechanism are perfectly suitable for thoracoscopy (Fig. 7). Disposable trocars are also available from several companies (Fig. 8). The insertion of curved instruments is only possible through flexible trocar tubes (Fig. 9).

5.2. Dissecting instruments

Many instruments are required: biopsy forceps, atraumatic grasping forceps, straight, curved and hooked scissors, etc. (Fig. 10). All these devices must be available in 3 versions: straight, right-curved and left-curved (Fig. 11). They can be connected to monopolar cautery. However, the intensive use of electrocautery may result in instrument tips being worn down quickly, especially scissor tips, so that disposable instruments are sometimes helpful (Fig. 12). Other dissecting instruments are also necessary, such as the dissector and coagulating hook.

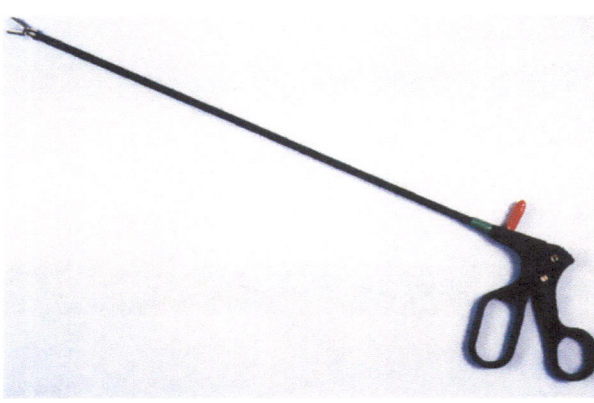

12

Fig. 12. Disposable grasping forceps (Ethicon)

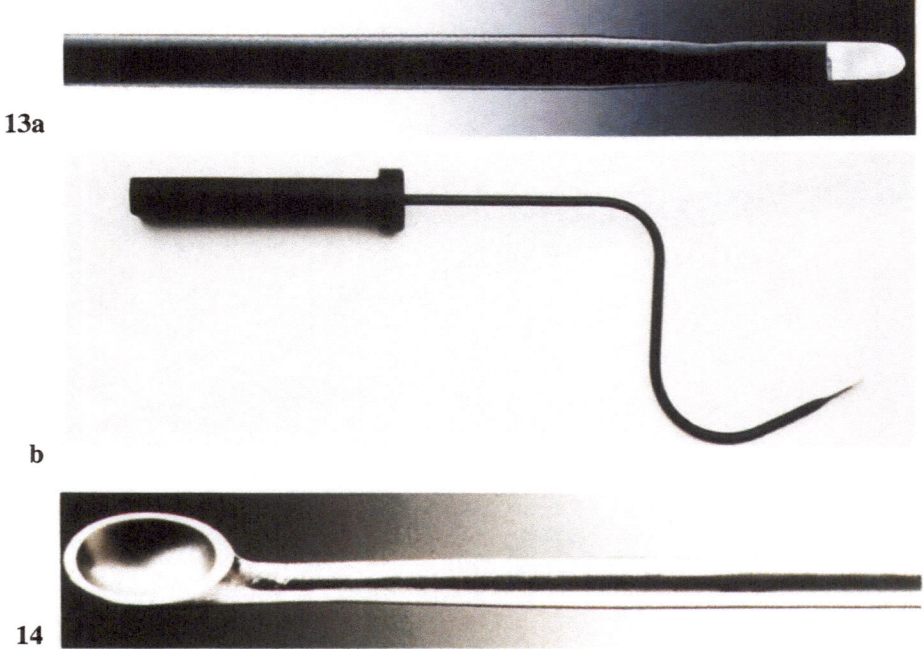

13a

b

Fig. 13a, b. Electrode spatulas : **a** straight and **b** double-curved (Olympus)

14

Fig. 14. Scraper for empyema debridement (Olympus)

5.3. Other instruments

- Spatulas are well adapted to pleurectomy. The double curved spatula makes it possible to begin pleural detachment around the puncture site (Fig. 13).

- Straight and curved suckers and scrapers are used in the treatment of hemothorax and debridement of empyemas (Fig. 14).

- Atraumatic lung forceps allow manipulation of pulmonary lobes. Esophageal forceps permit grasping the entire esophageal body and the performance of esophageal mobilisation.

- Several palpation probes and lung retractors are required, either narrow to flatten and explore the parenchyma, or broad to expose the posterior mediastinum and for efficient retraction of the lung.

- Disposable specimen retrieval bags are available from different companies (Fig. 15).

5.4. Suturing instrumentation

– The fact that entry sites need not to be air-tight makes it possible to introduce almost any type of needle, either through the trocar tube or directly through the

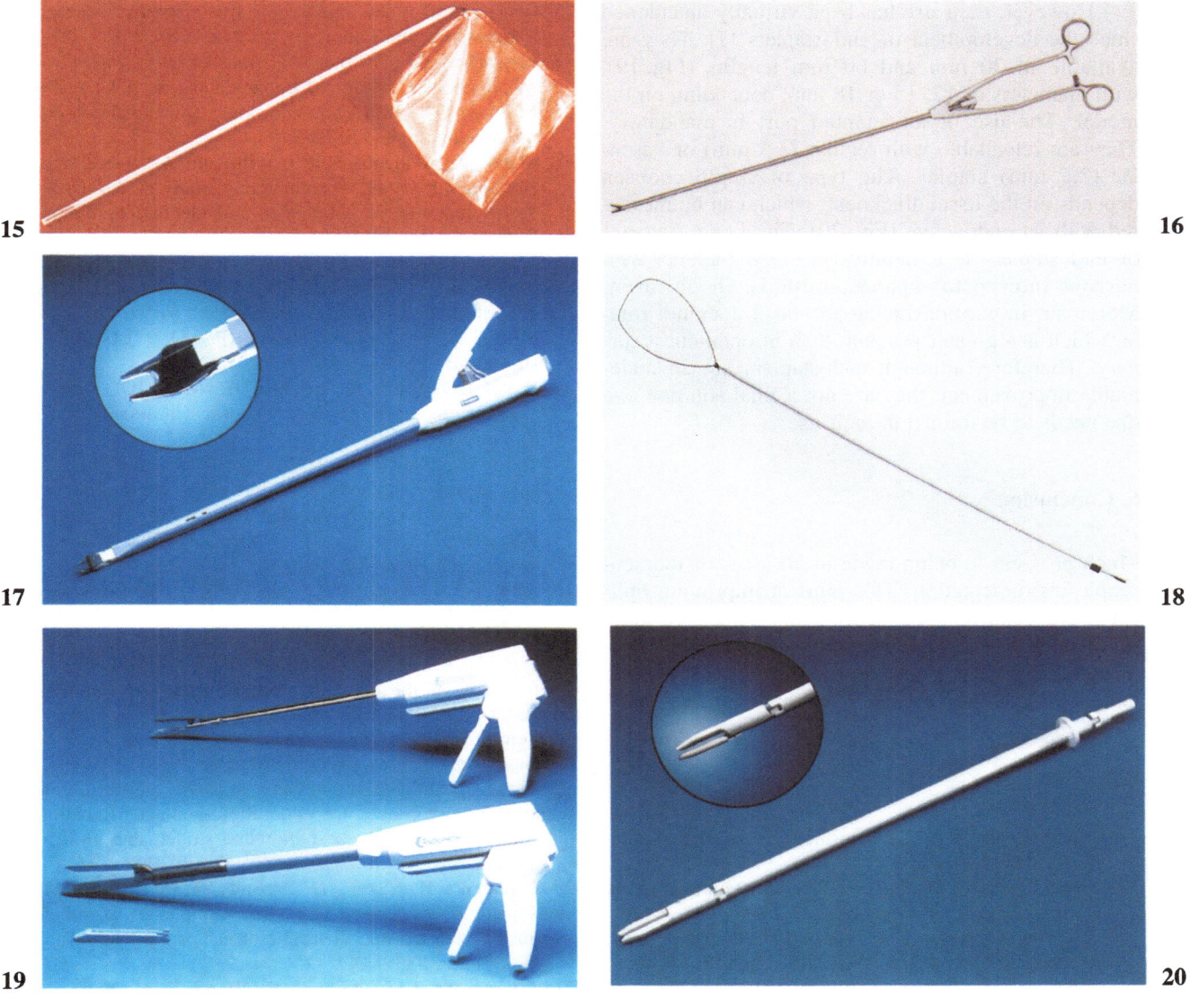

Fig. 15. Specimen retrieval bag (Ethicon)

Fig. 17. Clip applier (USSC)

Fig. 19. Endostaplers (Ethicon)

Fig. 16. Needle-holder (Olympus)

Fig. 18. Endo-Loop (Ethicon)

Fig. 20. Endogauge (USSC)

puncture opening. Few endoscopic needle-holders are as effective as the conventional ones; their jaws do not usually grasp the needle firmly enough, so that it is unstable. However, some titanium-reinforced needle-holders (Olympus) (Fig. 16) or needle-drivers with an internal piston mechanism (Cook) are efficient.

– Clips can be applied by disposable reloadable clip-appliers (Fig. 17). Some devices can apply different types of steel or absorbable clips.

– Ligation of vessels or pedicle blebs is possible with pre-tied endoscopic ligatures which are available in several suture materials (gut, polyglactin, polydioxanone) (Fig. 18).

– However, their use has been virtually abandoned since the development of endostaplers [7]. They are available in 30 mm and 60 mm lengths (Fig. 19), with diameters of 12, 15 or 18 mm, depending on the model. The use of an adapted port is mandatory. They are reloadable with regular (3.5 mm) or vascular (2,5 mm) staples. The type of staple choosen depends on the tissue thickness, which can be measured with an endogauge (Fig. 20). The large diameter of endostaplers is a liability in some patients with narrow intercostal spaces, notably in children. Moreover, in current models the head does not rotate, which is a greater problem than in open-chest surgery. Therefore, although endostaplers are an undeniable improvement, they are not a final solution and one needs to be trained in their use.

6. Conclusion

Much progress is being made in all areas of thoracoscopic instrumentation. This aims at improving optical quality and creating instruments which are more sophisticated and easier to manipulate. The development of flexible or semi-flexible telescopes with an integrated operating channel is perhaps the next step.

References

1. Boutin C (1989) The laser in thoracoscopy. Pneumologie 43 : 96-97
2. Boutin C, Viallat JR, Aleony Y (1990) Practical thoracoscopy. Springer-Verlag
3. Daikuzono N, Joffe SN (1985) Artificial sapphire probe for contact photocoagulation and tissue vaporization with the Nd. YAG laser. Med Instrum 19 : 173-178
4. Davidson AC, George RJ, Sheldon CD, Sinha G, Corrin B, Geddes DM (1988) Thoracoscopy assessment of a physician service and comparison of a flexible bronchoscope used as a thoracoscope with a rigid thoracoscope. Thorax 43 : 327-332
5. Ell C, Hochberger J (1987) Contact versus noncontact laser therapy. Gastrointest Endosc 33 : 125
6. Hunter JG (1991) Laser or electrocautery for laparoscopic cholecystectomy? Am J Surg 161 : 345-349
7. Krasna M, Nazen A (1991) Thoracoscopic lung resection : use of a new endoscopic linear stapler. Surgical Laparoscopy and Endoscopy 1 : 248-250
8. Lanzafame RJ (1990) Applications of lasers in laparoscopic cholecystectomy. J Laparoendosc Surg 1 : 33-36
9. Maassen W (1989) Thorakoskopie : Chirurgishe Technik. Pneumologie 43 : 53-54
10. Matek W, Reidenbach HD, Wittmann A, Beierlein L, Hermanek P (1989) A comparative study of the tissue-destroying effect of the laser and electrocoagulation. Endoscopy 21 : 31-36
11. Moghissi K, Deuch M, Goebells P (1988) Experience in non-contact Nd.YAG laser in pulmonary surgery. A pilot study Eur J Cardiothorac Surg 2 : 87-94
12. Murray A, Mitchell DC, Wood RFM (1991) Lasers in surgery. Br J Surg 79 : 21-26
13. Oakes DD, Sherk JP, Brodsky JB, Mark JDD (1984) Therapeutic thoracoscopy. J Thorac Cardiovasc Surg 87 : 269-273
14. Oldenburg FA, Newhouse MT (1979) Thoracoscopy : a safe, accurate diagnostic procedure using the rigid thoracoscope and local anesthesia. Chest 75 : 45-50
15. Rodgers BM, Moazam F, Talbert JL (1979) Thoracoscopy in children. Ann Surg 189 : 176-180
16. Sang CTM, Brainbridge MV (1981) Thoracoscopy simplified using the laparoscope. Thorac Cardiovasc Surgeon 29 : 129-130
17. Schroder R, Brackett K, Joffe SN (1987) An experimental study of the effects of electrocautery and various lasers on gastrointestinal tissue. Surgery 101 : 691-697
18. Semm K (1976) Endocoagulation : a new field of endoscopic surgery. J Reprod Med 16 : 175-180
19. Suzuki S, Shiina Y, Nomiyama T, Miwa T (1986) New ceramic endoprobes for endoscopic contact irradiation with Nd.YAG laser : experimental studies and clinical applications. Gastrointest Endosc 32 : 282-286
20. Tonotsuka H, Suzuki H, Akisawa T, Narushima M, Tanaka K, Kaneshiga H (1988) Intrapleural examinations by the flexible fiberoptic bronchoscope. Jp J Thorac Dis 26 : 936-942
21. Tsukamoto T, Nakamura H, Satoh T, Yamada K, Nagasawa M (1991) Comparative studies using a rigid thoracoscope and fiberoptic bronchoscope to treat spontaneaous pneumothorax. Chest 100 : 953-958
22. Unger SW, Arroyo P (1988) Nd. YAG laser applications in surgical endoscopy. A single center comprehensive experience. Am Surg 54 : 89-92
23. Wakabayashi A, Brenner M, Kayaleh RA, Berns MW, Barker SJ, Rice SJ, Tadir Y, Della Bella L, Wilson AF (1991) : Thoracoscopic carbon dioxide laser treatment of bullous emphysema. Lancet 337 : 881-883

Basic techniques in thoracoscopic surgery

D. Gossot

Thoracoscopic surgical techniques differ from open techniques in their instrumentation and the need for specialized videotechnique training. Although thoracoscopic operations are subject to the general principles of thoracic surgery, there are some significant differences between the endoscopic and the open approaches.

1. General considerations

Compared with thoracotomy, thoracoscopy has some advantages and some disadvantages.

A thoracoscopy offers the same view of the lung and mediastinum as a classic posterolateral thoracotomy and gives a better view of the lateral chest wall. Moreover, the field of vision is much better than in the small lateral incision which is often chosen for so-called minor procedures such as spontaneous pneumothorax treatment or benign tumor removal. Accurate dissection is facilitated by the videoendoscopic system's magnifying power. The cosmetic result is almost perfect and post-operative pain is minimal, due to the absence of chest-wall muscle division and rib-spreading. The only postoperative pain experienced is due to drainage and this disappears after the chest-tubes are removed. This minimal amount of pain in the post-operative course explains the low respiratory morbidity rate [15], a fact not yet demonstrated by randomised studies but obvious in clinical practice. As a result, the duration of hospitalisation can be reduced, as well as the need for postoperative physiotherapy.

Nevertheless, limitations for thoracoscopy do exist.

Manual palpation is not possible. This makes the localisation of small lung tumors almost impossible, unless they are peripheral and are visible on the parenchyma surface. This problem can be solved in part by using a small incision for finger insertion. In lung surgery the right dissection plane can not be found as easily as with the open technique in which one can feel the outline of a bronchus or perform manual peeling.

Endoscopic control of large vessels is theoretically possible. It has been shown in animal work, where the parenchyma is healthy, that pulmonary artery control is quite easy. However, in man, where vessels are often hindered and flattened by lymph-nodes or by a tumor, this control remains problematic and hazardous.

Thoracoscopy does not therefore have all the answers. It cannot be used in all cases and at the present time thoracotomy remains the standard approach for most major procedures.

Compared with other endoscopic techniques, surgical thoracoscopy has special features. The well known techniques used in laparoscopy cannot be applied as such in thoracoscopy. One of the main advantages of thoracoscopy is that insufflation is not needed and thus air leaks need not be dealt with. As a result, it is possible to combine thoracoscopy with an incision of several cm which allows the insertion of one or two fingers to palpate a nodule or to free any pleural adhesions before starting the endoscopic dissection (Fig. 21). An infant rib retractor can be used to spread the intercostal space [15]. In some ways, thoracoscopy is more difficult than laparoscopy. The manipulation of instruments is hindered by the rigidity of the chest and by the ribs and space is more limited, so that trocar location must be accurate and adapted to each procedure.

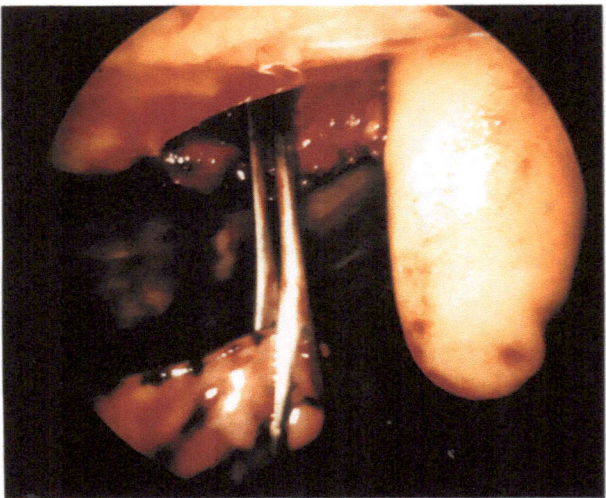

Fig. 21. A 3-5 cm incision allows insertion of conventional instruments and/or a finger for nodule palpation

2. Preparation

Diagnostic thoracoscopy in fragile patients can be performed under local anesthesia [11, 13] or local anesthesia completed by neuroleptanalgesia [1, 6]. But in all other cases, the operation must be performed under general anesthesia with tracheal intubation. Simple intubation is sufficient in some cases, such as for pleural effusion exploration, but it is usually better to have double lumen tracheal intubation [12]. Although the preoperative creation of a pneumothorax is recommended by most thoracoscopists [1, 5], it is not very useful, especially when the lung is collapsed through double-lumen tracheal intubation. The collapse can be completed by asking the anesthesist to aspirate the lung. The entry of air through the trocar tube helps to keep the lung collapsed so that, except in a few cases insufflation of the chest cavity is pointless [8]. Furthermore, it can be hazardous because of the potential risk of air embolism [14]. (During the procedure, the need for suction because of hemorrage or oozing causes an inflation of the lung which obstructs vision. This awkward phenomenon can be minimized by using many short suction periods instead of continuous aspiration and by leaving one or two ports empty.)

The same rules are applied as in conventional surgery. The draping is the same as for an open chest operation and the thoracotomy tray should be ready in the operating room.

Usually, the patient is in a lateral position [1, 7], although some authors prefer a supine position [2, 4] for all procedures. We find this position less convenient, the space for instrument manipulation being limited. Furthermore, in the supine position the lung does not deflate as much as in lateral position, thus limiting the field of vision (however, the supine position is indicated for some operations such as anterior mediastinal biopsies or pericardectomy). The operating table's bridge should be adjusted in the appropriate position but not elevated, unless the procedure is converted into an open one. Usually, it is more convenient to operate with the arm of the patient hanging down, because the manipulation of instruments can be hindered by the arm when the instruments tips are directed toward the lower part of the chest. However, in some procedures it is helpful to insert trocars in the axilla and then the arm must be elevated up. In overweight patients, it is useful to mark out the ribs with a pencil before starting the procedure. Generally, the surgeon is behind the patient's back, facing the TV monitor.

3. Trocar insertion

The first 10 mm-trocar is introduced into the 5th, 6th or 7th intercostal space (ICS), depending on the procedure to be performed. The incision is made at the upper border of the rib, using a sharp scalpel. The trocar path is created with smooth forceps until the pleura is identified. The pleura is opened unless an extrapleural approach is chosen [7]. Thorough hemostasis of the trocar path avoids any unpleasant oozing along the trocar sheath. The round-tip trocar is gently introduced, a smooth tip being mandatory in order to avoid lung trauma in cases with unexpected pleural adhesions. The other ports are introduced using the same technique, under video control. The precise location of the additional ports must be marked out by depressing the ICS with a finger or forceps tip, or by introducing a needle in the ICS.

4. Endoscope

The telescope must be inserted remote from the lesion and from the operative field, and in a position opposite to them [1]. For instance, in a posteriorinferior empyema, the best endoscope location would be in the 5th ICS, in the anterior axillary line. The use of a 30° telescope helps to reduce the dead angle (Fig. 22). Another way to examine almost all of the chest cavity is to change the endoscope insertion

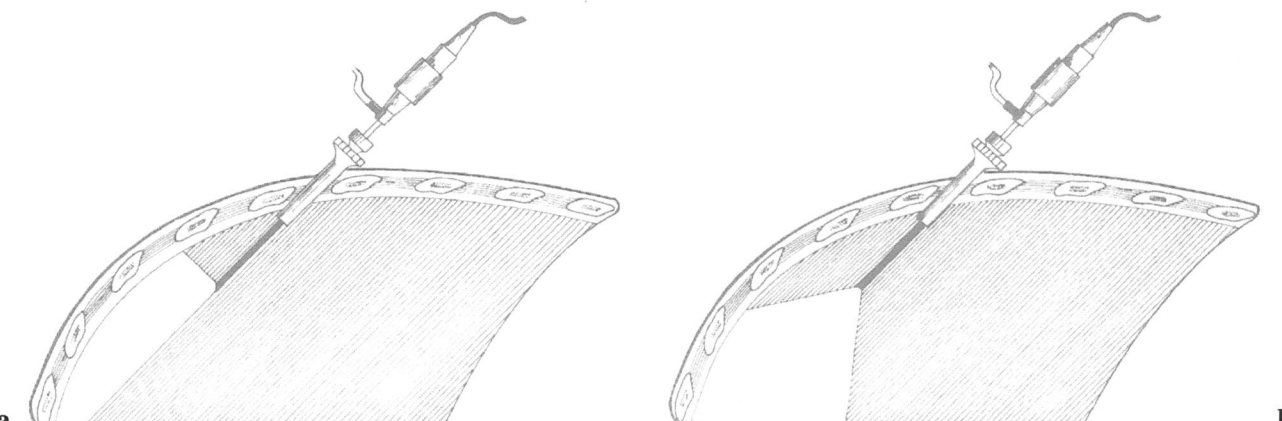

Fig. 22a, b. Comparison of the fields of vision offered by **a** a 0° telescope and **b** a 30° telescope. The 30° telescope reduces the dead angle

during the procedure, from the anterior to the posterior axillary line. In the case of an extrapleural approach, a double control can be used with an extrapleural and an endopleural endoscope [7].

During the thoracoscopic procedure the vision is often blurred by blood drops on the scope, sliding down along the trocar tube. Cleaning the small thoracoscopic trocar sheath is easily accomplished with the use of sterile cotton-tips. Vision can also be hampered by fog. This problem can be solved by the use of a telescope heater or by the application of hot serum or a drop of chlorhexidine on the telescope tip.

5. Instruments

The instruments are introduced through a 5 or a 10 mm trocar tube according to their diameter and through rigid or flexible trocars according to their shape. Although it is possible to manipulate the instruments without a trocar tube, this must be avoided because the rib edge damages the instrument sheath. In addition, the direct insertion of instruments without a trocar tube increases the risk of an intercostal vessel injury.

In order to have sufficient control of the instruments, they must be introduced remote from the telescope (Fig. 23). The use of curved instruments makes many manipulations much easier, because it enlarges their field of action and allows them to reach some areas which straight devices cannot

(Fig. 24). The benefit of curved instruments has been demonstrated in other endoscopic procedures [3, 10].

Because of the long shape of the chest, the dissection of some upper mediastinal structures may be difficult with instruments inserted at the lower chest. In this case, one should make additional entry sites for both endoscope and dissecting tools in front of the structure to be dissected. This permits more control by avoiding an awkward tangential view. These multiple punctures have a minimal cosmetic drawback, and do not impair postoperative respiratory function or increase postoperative pain.

6. Suturing techniques

The need for suturing is not usual with current thoracoscopic procedures. However, unexpected situations may be encountered, such as a defect between two rows of staples or a lung injury requiring suture. The absence of air-leak problems in thoracoscopy means that simpler techniques can be used than in laparoscopy. The needle can be introduced either in the trocar tube or without a tube, directly through the puncture site, if the needle is too large.

6.1. Continuous suture

The suture line is cut to the desired length. A clip is applied at the end opposite to the needle and is firmly tightened (Fig. 25a, c) The continuous suture is made using an endoscopic needleholder and a gras-

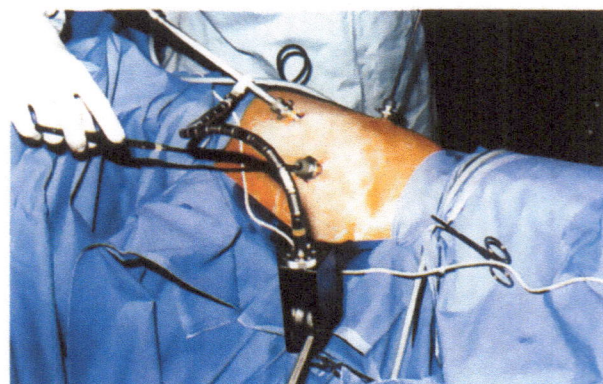

Fig. 23. Usual triangulation position of manual instruments and telescope

Fig. 24. a Curved instruments can reach areas which cannot be reached by **b** straight instruments

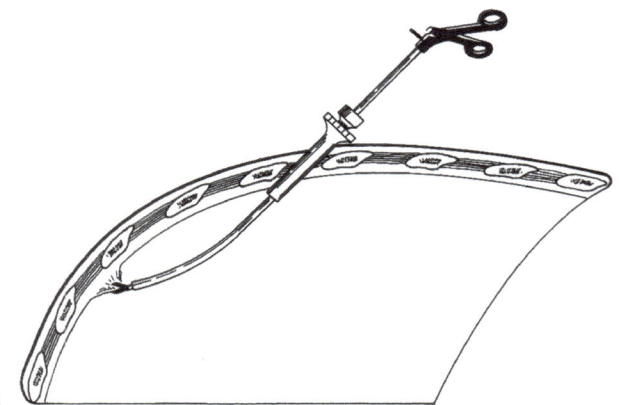

24a

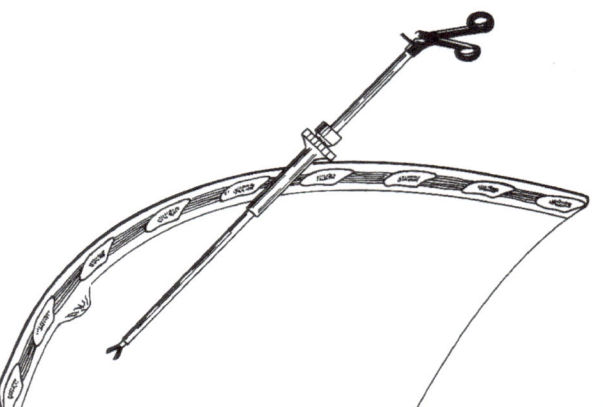

b

per. The function of the grasper is to present the needle in the right position in relation to the needle-holder, to grasp the needle when it has passed through the tissue and to control tension on the suture as it is drawn through the tissue. It also helps to depress the tissue at the anticipated needle exit point should the needle tip be too difficult to see. This provides a better exposure of the needle (Fig. 25b) When the continuous suture is finished, it is fastened off with a clip and cut (Fig. 25d) This technique allows for a suture line of only a few centimeters, thus making the manipulation easier.

6.2. Interrupted suture

Numerous techniques of knot tying have been described, including intracorporeal and extracorporeal procedures.

The intracorporeal technique requires intensive training and practice, but has few indications in sur-

gical thoracoscopy. It is possible to tie almost all the sutures outside the chest. The needle is introduced into the chest. The opposite end of the thread, remaining through the trocar sheath, can be secured outside the chest with a forceps to avoid its accidental sliding into the operative field. The needle is passed through the tissue as previously described, then withdrawn through the trocar tube (Fig. 26a). A single-throw knot is made with the two suture ends (Fig. 26b). This knot is held with the thumb and second finger (Fig. 26c). With the free end of the suture, three revolutions are made around both suture strands (Fig. 26d). The tail of the suture is inserted through the first loop and then through the loop that was formed below the initial single-throw knot. The tail is pulled up and cut. By simply pulling the end of the thread, the knot slides down by itself. It is then pushed with a knot tier or an atraumatic forceps and secured (Fig. 26e). Finally, the suture is cut off 3 mm from the knot (Fig. 26f).

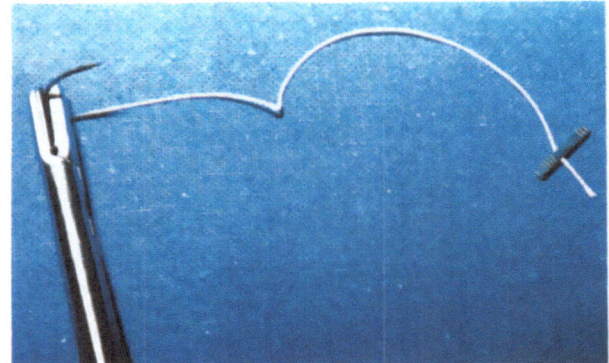

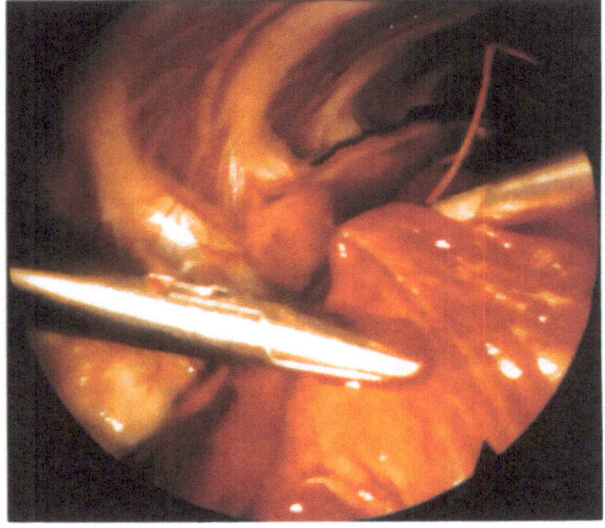

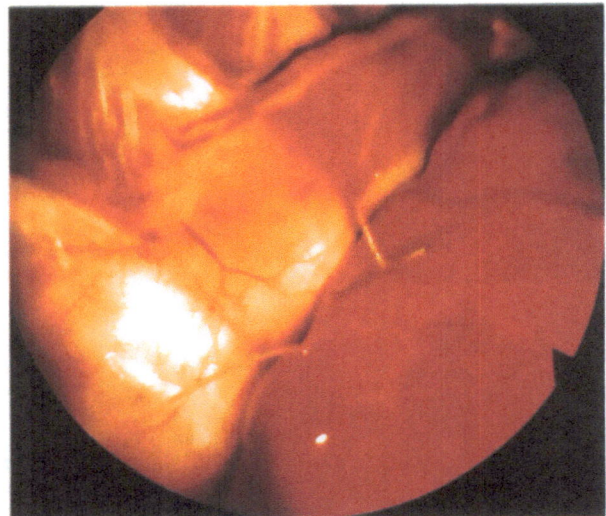

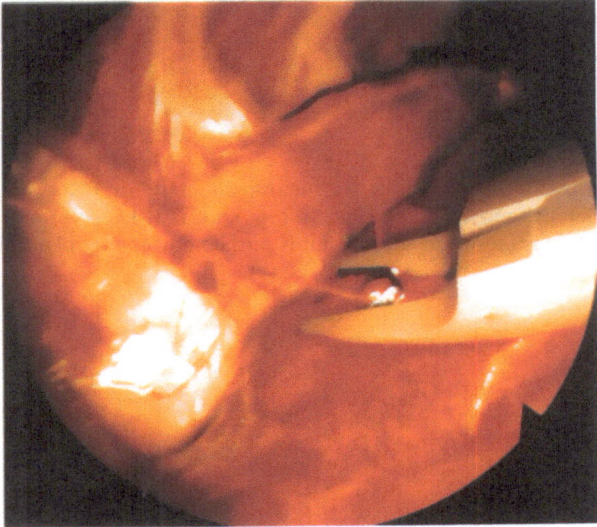

Fig. 25a-d. Technique for continuous suture. **a** A clip is applied and tightened at the end of a 10-12 cm wire. **b** Using a grasper or a second needle holder helps to expose the needle. **c** View of the first suture. **d** The continuous suture is finished and fastened with a clip

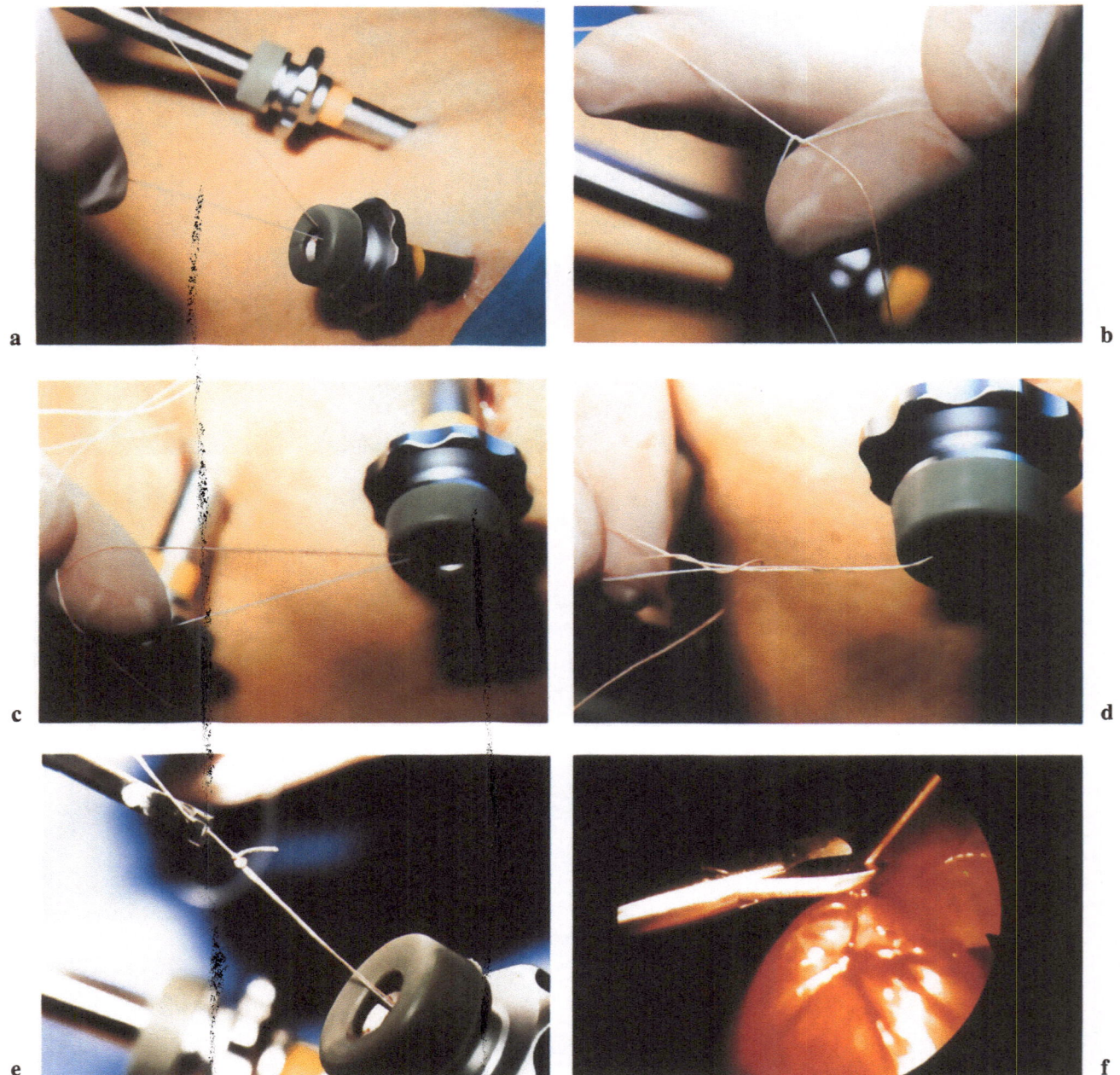

Fig. 26a-f. Technique for interrupted suture. **a** The two ends are withdrawn through the trocar tube. **b** A single-throw knot is made. **c** The single-throw knot is held with the thumb and the second finger. **d** Three revolutions around both strands are made. **e** The knot is pushed down with a knot-tier. **f** The suture is finished and cut

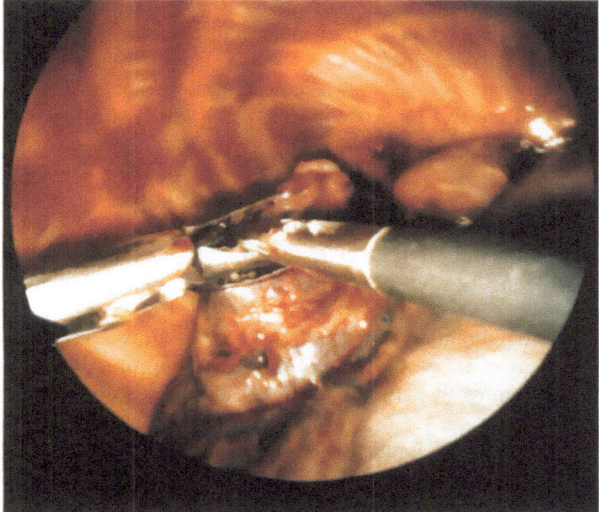

27a

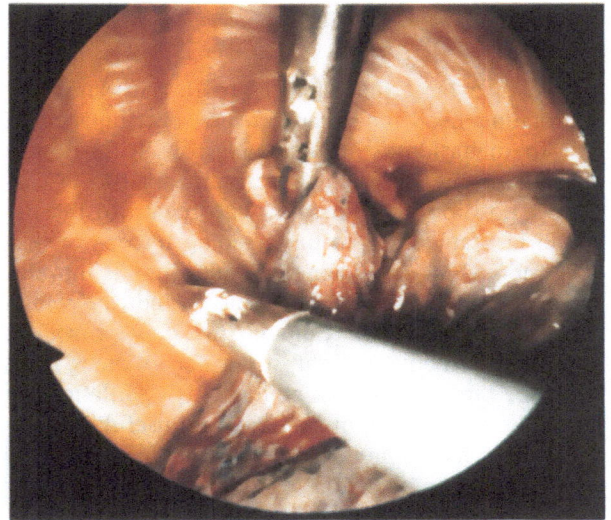

b

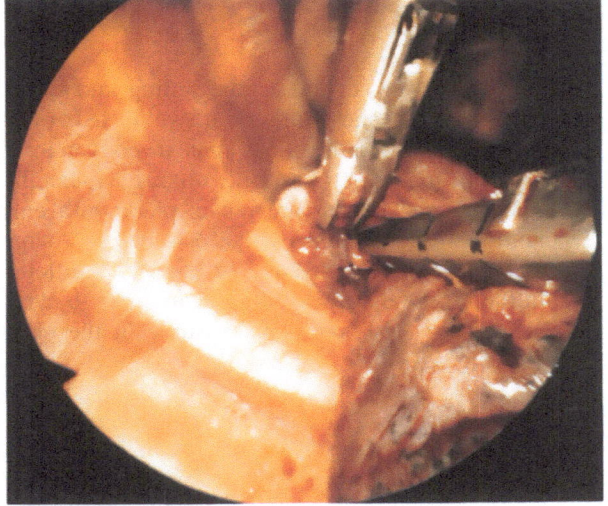

c

Fig. 27a-c. Stapling technique (example: excision of a bleb). **a** The parenchyma is grasped with a forceps. Before introducing the stapler, its direction is tested with a 5 mm device. In this case, the direction is not correct: the two instruments are crossed. **b** The position of the forceps has been changed. The 5 mm-device indicates that the direction of the stapler will be correct. **c** The stapler can be applied

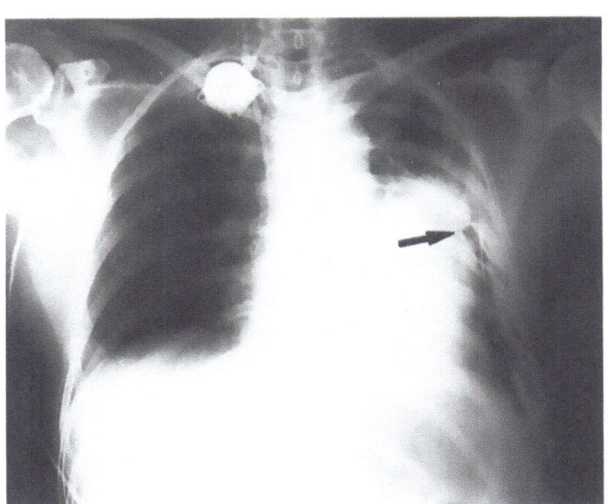

Fig. 28. Kinking of a chest tube *(arrow)*, whose position was not endoscopically controlled

28

7. Stapling techniques

Due to their large diameter (12 to 18 mm) and their nonrotating head, endostaplers are sometimes difficult to manipulate through a narrow ICS. Before introducing the stapler, it is recommended to test its correct position and direction with regard to the tissue to be stapled and to the grasping forceps, with a 5 mm tool (Fig. 27). Then, the endogauge is introduced and clamped on to the tissue to indicate which staple size to choose. Although the staple rows are generally perfectly air-tight, it is safer to check them by saline serum irrigation while gently ventilating the lung. The oversewing of staples is not useful.

Specific techniques of endoscopic lung stapling are described on page 76.

8. Chest drainage

The same principles of chest tube setting and management as in open chest surgery are valid. It is often possible to insert smaller tubes than in conventional surgery, because postoperative oozing is usually reduced. If 2 chest tubes are put in place with only 2 puncture sites, the first is placed under videocontrol, but the second is inserted in blindly. The latter should therefore be a trocar catheter in order to avoid a false passage or kinking of the tube in the chest wall [9] (Fig. 28).

References

1. Boutin C, Viallat JR, Aelony Y (1990) Practical Thoracoscopy. Springer-Verlag
2. Byrne J, Walsh TN, Hederman WP (1990) Endoscopic transthoracic electrocautery of the sympathetic chain for palmar and axillary hyperhidrosis. Br J Surg 77 : 1046-1049
3. Cushieri A (1991) Variable curvature shape-memory spatula for laparoscopic surgery. Surg Endosc 5 : 179-181
4. Daniel TM, Curtis GT, Rodgers BM (1990) Thoracoscopy and talc poudrage for pneumothoraces and effusions. Ann Thorac Surg 50 : 186-189
5. Faurschou P (1984) Induction of pneumothorax by means of the Veres cannula. Eur J Resp Dis 65 : 547-549
6. Gillet-Juvin K, Guérin JC (1991) Le talcage sous thoracoscopie des pneumothorax par rupture de bulles d'emphysème. Étude de 71 cas. Rev Mal Resp 8 : 289-293
7. Levi JF, Kleinmann Ph, Riquet M, Debesse B (1990) Percutaneous parietal pleurectomy for recurrent spontaneous pneumothorax. Lancet 336 : 1577-1578
8. Maassen W (1981) Thoracoscopie et biopsie pulmonaire sans pneumothorax initial. Poumon-Coeur 37 : 317-319
9. Miller KS, Sahn SA (1987) Chest tubes. Indications, techniques, management and complications. Chest 91 : 258-264
10. Nathanson LK, Shimi S, Cushieri A (1991) Laparoscopic ligamentum teres cardiopexy. Br J Surg 78 : 947-951
11. Oldenburg FA Jr, Newhouse MT (1979) Thoracoscopy : a safe, accurate diagnostic procedure, using the rigid thoracoscope and local anesthesia. Chest 75 : 45-50
12. Page RD, Jeffrey RR, Donnelly RJ (1989) Thoracoscopy : a review of 121 consecutive surgical procedures. Ann Thorac Surg 48 : 66-68
13. Vanderschuren RG (1981) Thoracoscopie sous anesthésie locale. Poumon-Coeur 37 : 55-515
14. Viskum K (1989) Contraindications and complications to thoracoscopy. Pneumologie 43, 55-57
15. Wakabayashi A (1991) Expanded applications of diagnostic and therapeutic thoracoscopy. J Thorac Cardiovasc Surg 102 : 721-723

Anesthesia for thoracoscopy

N.S. Trivedi and S.J. Barker

In recent years, there has been renewed interest in thoracoscopy, both as a diagnostic as well as a therapeutic procedure. Thoracoscopy is greatly facilitated by collapsing the operated lung and ventilating the non-operated lung (one lung ventilation). Wakabayashi reports that therapeutic laser thoracoscopy is widely used in patients with severely compromised cardio-pulmonary functions. The anesthetic management of these patients is very challenging. With the recent advances in invasive monitoring, newer and safer anesthetic agents, and a better understanding of the pathophysiology of cardiopulmonary diseases, the anesthetic management of these patients is now possible.

At the present time, thoracoscopy is mainly performed for the following diagnostic and therapeutic indications:

– Diagnostic indications: pleural biopsy of lung tumor, mediastinal lymph node biopsy and biopsy of mediastinal mass.

– Therapeutic indications: debridement and pleurectomy for pleural effusion, ablation of pseudopneumocysts in the treatment of spontaneous pneumothorax, laser bullectomy for diffuse bullous emphysema, debridement of acute and chronic empyema, sympathectomy and truncal vagotomy, pericardial window. Other major procedures have recently been described such as lung resection including segmentectomy as well as lobectomy and esophagectomy.

All these procedures require thoroughly pre-operative evaluation.

1. Pre-operative evaluation

The pre-operative evaluation goals for patients undergoing thoracoscopy are as follows: to assess the extent of primary disease and associated medical problems, to optimize the medical status of the patient and to understand perioperative management problems.

The pre-operative evaluation should include:

– A routine laboratory work up: CBC, electrolytes, BUN, creatinine, liver function tests and urine analysis.

– Coagulation profile.

– Electro cardiogram [EKG].

– Chest X-ray and CT-scan in some cases.

– Pulmonary function tests [PFTs] including: Forced Expiratory Volume in one seconde [FEV1], Functional Vital Capacity [FVC], FEV1/FVC, Residual Volume/Total Lung Capacity [RV/CPT] and Arterial Blood Gas [ABG].

The pre-operative PFTs may reveal an increase operative risk. Preoperative pulmonary factors are summarized below:

– *Spirometry and ABG:*

• FEV1/FVC : < 50%

• FEV1 : < 2 liters (L)

• RV/TLC : > 50%

• Hypercapnia/hypoxemia at room air temperature.

– *Split lung function:*

• FEV1 < 0.85 L.

• More than 70% blood flow to the diseased lung.

– *Balloon occlusion of pulmonary artery [PA]:*

• Mean Pulmonary Artery Pressure [PAP] > 40 mmHg.

• PCO2 > 60 mmHg.

• PO2 < 45 mmHg.

2. Intra-operative monitoring

For standard diagnostic procedures, a routine monitoring is used. It includes a five lead EKG with analysis of the ST segment, a pulse oximetry to measure oxygen saturation, a transcutaneous 02 measurement indicating 02 tension at tissue level, a capnography to monitor adequate ventilation, a urine output to monitor renal function and volume status and a temperature monitoring.

In fragile patients or in case of major procedure, a more invasive monitoring is recommended. Two blood lines should be used: one 14 G peripheral IV for volume resuscitation and one 20 G radial arterial line for continuous blood pressure monitoring as well as frequent measurements of ABG, electrolytes and hematocrit. A CVP/PA catheter permits measurements of continous mixed venous oxygen saturation, PA pressures and cardiac output.

3. Anesthetic management

Many patients undergoing thoracoscopy have poor cardio-pulmonary functions and may have not been able to tolerate any pre-medication. An informational interview with the patient usually reduces anxiety significantly. When the patient is brought to the operating room, invasive line placement is performed under local anesthesia. During this period, light seda-tion may be administered as tolerated. Following adequate pre-oxygenation, induction of anesthesia is achieved using high doses of potent narcotics (Sufentanil/Fentanyl). Narcotic induction provides good hemodynamic stability. Muscle relaxation is adequately achieved while maintaining hemodynamic stability by using non-depolarizing muscle relaxant (e.g Vecuronium). Maintenance of anesthesia is achieved with narcotics and/or inhalation anesthetics.

Thoracoscopy requires one lung ventilation (OLV) which is easily performed using a Robert-Shaw double lumen endobronchial tube (DLT). Left sided DLT is usually preferred for a surgical procedure on either the right or left lung, because placement of a left DLT is less difficult. The placement of a right DLT is difficult, because the right upper lobe bronchus origin is close to the carina. If the distal orifice on the right DLT is not placed at the origin of right upper lobe (RUL) bronchus, ventilation of RUL is compromised, leading to atelectasis and hypoxemia (Fig. 29).

Placement of the DLT is confirmed by:
– Chest wall movements.
– Presence of mist.
– Auscultation of breath sounds when one of the lumens is blocked.
– Fiberoptic bronchoscopy:
• For a left DLT, look for the margin of the blue cuff just below the carina on the left side.
• For a right DLT, ensure that the RUL bronchus origin matches the distal orifice on the right DLT (Fig. 30).

Double-Lumen Tubes

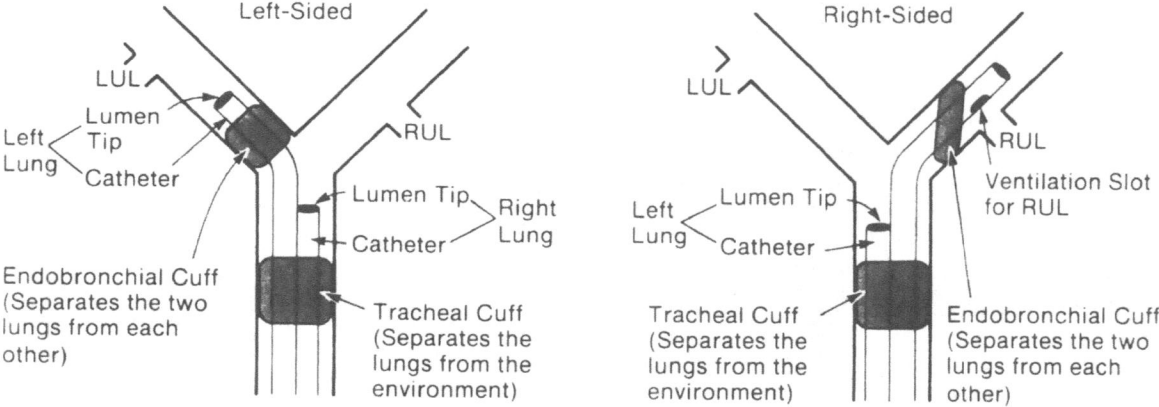

Fig. 29. This diagram explains the essential features and parts of the Right sided and Left sided double lumen endobronchial tubes. RUL = Right Upper Lobe, LUL = Left Upper Lobe (with permission: Benumof JL, Anesthesia for Thoracic Surgery, 1987, WB Saunders Company, Philadelphia)

Use of Fiberoptic Bronchoscope to Determine
Precise Right-Sided Double-Lumen Tube Position

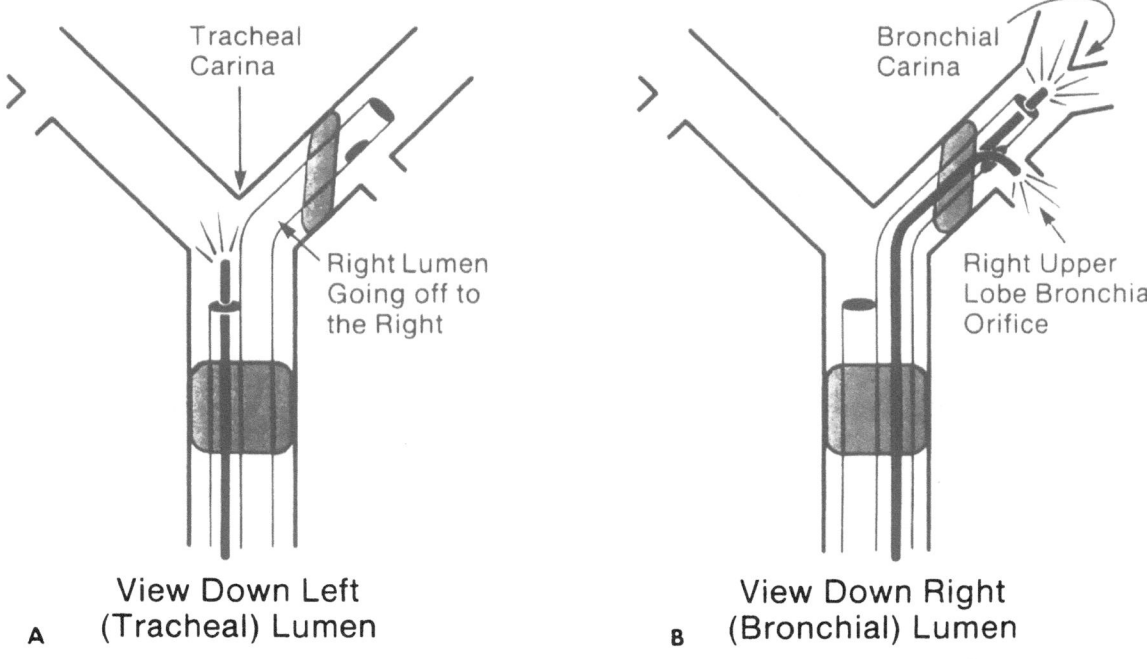

A   **View Down Left**
(Tracheal) Lumen

B   **View Down Right**
(Bronchial) Lumen

Fig. 30A, B. This diagram explains the use of a fiberoptic bronchoscope to determine precise right-sided double lumen tube position. **A** When a fiberoptic bronchoscope is passed down the tracheal lumen, a clear straight-ahead view of tracheal carina and the right lumen going off into the right mainstem bronchus is obtained. **B** When the fiberoptic bronchoscope is passed down the bronchial lumen, the bronchial carina is seen off in the distance. When the fiberoptic bronchoscope is flexed cephalad and passed through the right upper lobe ventilation slot, the right upper lobe bronchial orifice should be visualised (with permission: Benumof JL, Anesthesia for Thoracic Surgery, 1987, WB Saunders Company, Philadelphia)

3.1. One lung ventilation

One lung ventilation is mandatory to provide a quiet surgical field during thoracoscopy. For therapeutic thoracoscopy, it is required for a prolonged period of time (120-180 min) and is achieved by using a Robert-Shaw DLT. When one lung ventilation is required, the lumen ventilating the operated lung is clamped, thus no ventilation takes place in that. Once one lung ventilation begins, a tidal volume of 10 ml/kg is maintained and the respiratory rate is adjusted to maintain a $PCO_2 < 40$ mmHg. Aggressive monitoring of frequent ABGs, ventilation and cardiovascular status are essential. Even minor hemodynamic changes should be treated aggressively. Hypoxemia and large air leaks are two major problems which may be experienced during thoracoscopy.

3.1.1. Management of hypoxemia

When PaO_2 falls below 70 mmHg, a diagnosis of hypoxemia should be considered, warranting aggressive management:

– Check the position of the DLT with fiberoptic bronchoscopy.

– Check the patient's hemodynamic status and treat any changes aggresively.

– Increase FIO2.

– Add CPAP [5-10 cm] to non-dependent lung, i.e upper non-ventilated lung.

– Add PEEP [5-15 cm] to dependent lung, i.e lower ventilated lung.

– CPAP/PEEP search as per Benumof is effective (Fig. 31).

– In case of persistant hypoxemia, use intermittent two lung ventilation.

A ONE LUNG VENTILATION: THE SITUATION   **B** ONE LUNG VENTILATION: DOWN LUNG PEEP

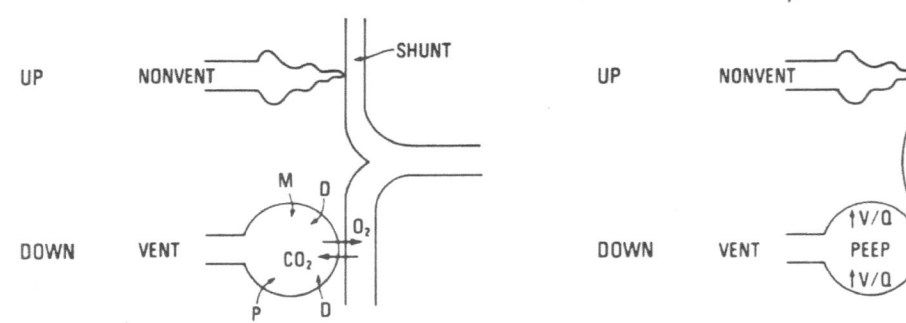

C ONE LUNG VENTILATION: UP LUNG CPAP   **D** ONE LUNG VENTILATION: DIFFERENTIAL LUNG $\frac{CPAP}{PEEP}$

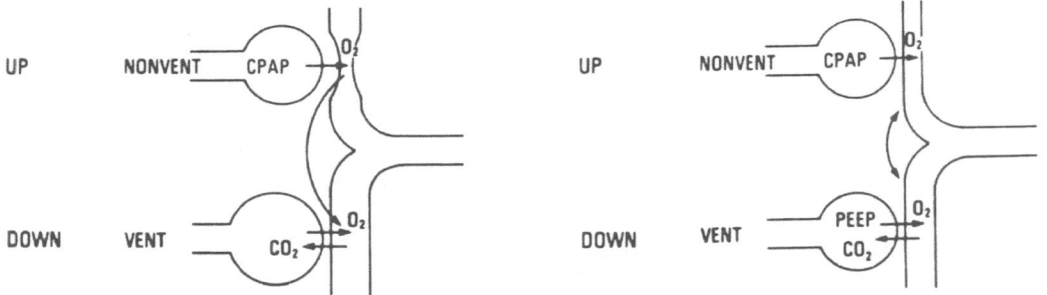

Fig. 31A-D. This diagram shows effects of various differential lung management approaches in four parts. **A** The one lung ventilation [OLV]: the dependent lung [down] is ventilated but is compressed by weight of mediastinum [M] from above, the pressure of the abdominal contents against the diaphragm [D] and by positioning effect of rolls, packs and shoulder support [P]. The nondependent [UP] lung is not ventilated and the blood flow through this lung is shunt flow. **B** OLV: Down lung PEEP. The dependent lung has been selectively treated with PEEP which improves the ventilation to perfusion [V/Q] relationship in the dependent lung but also increases the dependent lung vascular resistance. This diverts blood to up lung which increases the shunt flow. **C** OLV: Up lung CPAP. Selective application of continuous positive airway pressure [CPAP] to the up lung permits the oxygen uptake from this lung. Even if CPAP causes an increase in vascular resistance, the diverted blood flow can still participate in gas exchange in the ventilated lung. Consequently, selective nondependent lung CPAP can greatly increase PaO2. **D** OLV: Differential lungs CPAP/PEEP. With differential lung CPAP [nondependent lung] and PEEP [dependent lung] both lung can participate in O2 uptake and oxygenation can be achieved to levels near to those achieved by two lung ventilation (with permission: in Miller RD, Anesthesia, 3rd Edition, 1990 Thoracic Anesthesia, Benunof JL, Alfrey DD, Churchill Livingstone, New York)

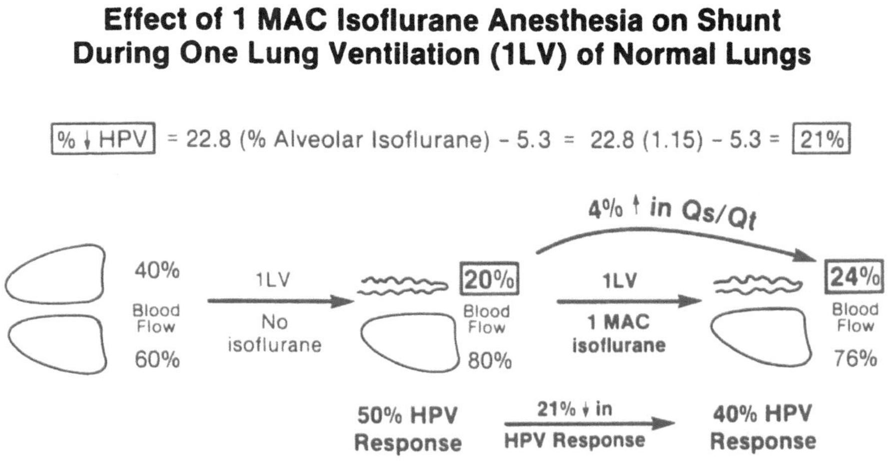

Effect of 1 MAC Isoflurane Anesthesia on Shunt During One Lung Ventilation (1LV) of Normal Lungs

$\boxed{\% \downarrow \text{HPV}}$ = 22.8 (% Alveolar Isoflurane) − 5.3 = 22.8 (1.15) − 5.3 = $\boxed{21\%}$

Fig. 32. This diagram shows the theoretical distribution of the blood flow between the nondependent and dependent lungs for patients with normal lungs for two lungs ventilation, one lung ventilation and one lung ventilation with 1 MAC Isoflurane anesthesia (with permission: Benunof JL: Anesthesiology V 64, N° 4, 1986)

– If all else fails, use two lung ventilation.

During two lung ventilation in lateral decubitus position, non-dependent [upper] lung receives 40% of pulmonary blood flow while dependent [lower] lung receives 60% of pulmonary blood flow. When the ventilatory pattern is changed to one lung ventilation, hypoxic pulmonary vasoconstriction [HPV] response occurs in the non-dependent lung, decreasing blood flow by 50%. So, the non-dependent/dependent lung blood flow ratio becomes 20%/80%. Even with HPV, there may be hypoxemia. During OLV if patient receives 1 MAC [1.15%] of isoflurane, HPV response decreases by 21% [40% instead of 50%].

Consequently, the nondependent/dependent lung blood flow ratio would now become 24%/76%, representing a 4% increase in the total shunt across the lungs, which may worsen hypoxemia. This phenomenon is described on Figure 32.

3.1.2. Management of large air-leak

Following therapeutic treatment of bullous disease, it is not uncommon to have large air leaks. When the air leak is greater than 50%,

$$\left(\frac{\text{Inspired Tidal Volume} - \text{Expired Tidal Volume}}{\text{Inspired Tidal Volume}} \times 100 \right)$$

it must be corrected surgically. Volume ventilators are not very effective in achieving adequate minute ventilation with air leaks. Pressure controlled ventilators, i.e Siemens Servo 900 C, are very effective in delivering the desired tidal volume and adequate minute ventilation.

4. Post-operative course

Following thoracoscopy, the DLT should be changed in the operating room to a large size single lumen endotracheal tube. Post-operative ventilation is maintained adequately by using a pressure controlled ventilator, with adequate minute ventilation to maintain normocapnia. PEEP should not be used, as this may lead to increased air leak. In case early extubation has been unsuccessful, mechanical ventilatory support should be continued for a prolonged period. These patients benefit from post-operative pain control administrated through PCA or thoracic epidural analgesia.

References

1. Anderson HW, Benumof JL (1981) Intrapulmonary shunting during one-lung ventilation and surgical manipulation. Anesthesiology 55 : 377
2. Benumof JL (1979) Hypoxemic pulmonary vasoconstriction and infusion of sodium nitroprusside (Editorial). Anesthesiology 50 : 481-483
3. Benumof JL (1986) Isoflurane Anesthesia and arterial oxygenation during one lung ventilation. Anesthesiology 64 : 419-424

4. Benumof JL (1987) Anesthesia for Thoracic Surgery. Philadelphia, WB Saunders, pp 227-285

5. Casthely PA, Lear S, Cottrell JE, Lear E (1985) Intrapulmonary shunting during induced hypotension. Anesth Anal 61 : 231-235.

6. Chubra-Smith NM, Grant RP, Jenkins LC (1986) Perioperative transcutaneous oxygen monitoring in thoracic anesthesia. Can Anaesth Soc J 33 : 745-753

7. Dantzker DR, Wagner PD, West JB (1975) Instability of lung with low VA/Q rations during oxygen breathing. J App 1 Physiol 38 : 886-895

8. Kerr JH, Crampton-Smith A, Prys-Robert C, Meloche R, Foex P (1974) Observations during endobronchial anesthesia II: Oxygenation. Br J Anaesth 46 : 84-92

9. Miller RD (1990) Anesthesia Third Edition, Chap 50, Anesthesia for Thoracic Surg, pp 1517-1603

10. Page RD, Jeffery RR, Donnelly RJ (1989) Thoracoscopy: A review of 121 consecutive surgical procedures. Ann Thorac Surg 48 : 66-68

11. Piper P, Vane J (1971) The release of Prostaglandins form lung and other tissues. Ann NY Acad Sci 180 : 363-385.

12. Ray JF, Vost L, Moallem S, Sanoudos GM, Villamena P, Parades RM, Claus RH (1974) Immobility, hypoxemia and pulmonary arteriovenous shunting. Arch Surg 109 : 537-541

13. Trempor KK, Barker SJ (1987) Transcutaneous oxygen mesurement: Experimental studies and adult applications. Int Anesth Clinics 3 : 73

14. Wakabayashi A (1989) Thoracoscopic ablation of blebs in the treatment of recurent or persistent spontaneous pneumothorax. Ann Thorac Surg 48 : 651-653

The role of thoracoscopy in the diagnosis of pleural pathology

J. Bourcereau and N. Gharbi

1. Introduction

Diagnostic difficulties in pleural disorders have given rise to several studies [1-7]. But such problems still exist in everyday practice. In addition to the sensitivities and specificities of the various examinations two other aspects must be taken into account. The first concerns emergencies, which are not only dictated by respiratory difficulty but also by the patient himself, who expects a rapid solution to his problem. The second aspect involves exploratory procedures, which must be the minimally harmful and costly.

There are four types of pleural pathology with distinct pathogenic forms but with similar clinical aspects (i.e. dominated by dyspnea and thoracic pain). They are as follows: pneumothorax, hydropneumothorax, pleural tumor, and pleural effusion. The same etiology may be responsible for one or more of these clinical types. This is explained physiopathologically [8-13]. Knowledge of the anatomy and physiology of the pleura leads to an understanding of its pathology and the development of the necessary diagnostic methods necessary.

Iatrogenic pleural pathology, spontaneous pneumothorax in young patients and pneumothorax as a complication in an older emphysematous patient create few problems in diagnosis. Apart from these cases, the diagnostic process in pleural pathology must follow a "decisional algorithm" regardless of the causative disorder. The description of this practical algorithm constitutes the aim of this study.

2. Pleural pathology without pleurisy

A diagnosis must be made in the presence of either more or less significant dyspnea of recent appearance, or a parietal type of pain limiting respiration or lastly, a radiographic abnormality discovered fortuitously. According to whether pleural effusion is present or not, two orientations are distinguished from each other (Fig. 33).

In the absence of effusion a pneumothorax may be involved complicating either a pulmonary or pleural tumor, or as a result of the rupture of a mediastinal structure. Diagnosis is made as in all tumoral or traumatic thoracic pathology.

Radiographs of the thorax, thoracic and/or abdominal CT-scans, tracheobronchial endoscopy and if necessary esophagoscopy permit making the diagnosis, which calls for histologic confirmation in cases of tumor. Biopsy is made using transparietal or thoracoscopic procedures. A benign pleural tumor may be involved such as fibroma, associated in some cases with abnormal secretion of an insulin-like hormone [14-16]. In other instances a malignant primary or secondary tumor may be present. The most representative tumor is the mesothelioma in which the history and the patient's occupational career may point to a causal association with asbestos.

3. Pleural pathology with pleurisy

In the presence of a pleural effusion, associated or not with a pleural, pulmonary, or mediastinal tumor, other steps may be envisaged (Fig. 34). The clinical picture, radiographic aspects, CT-scans and ultrasound examinations permit evaluation of the fluid volume and degree of pleural involvement and guide the diagnostic process.

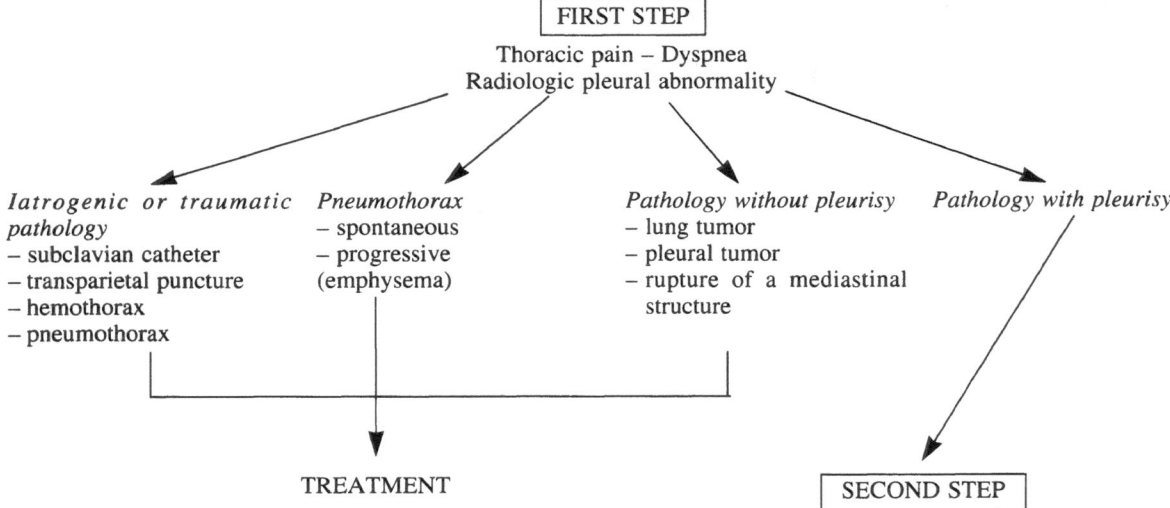

Fig. 33.

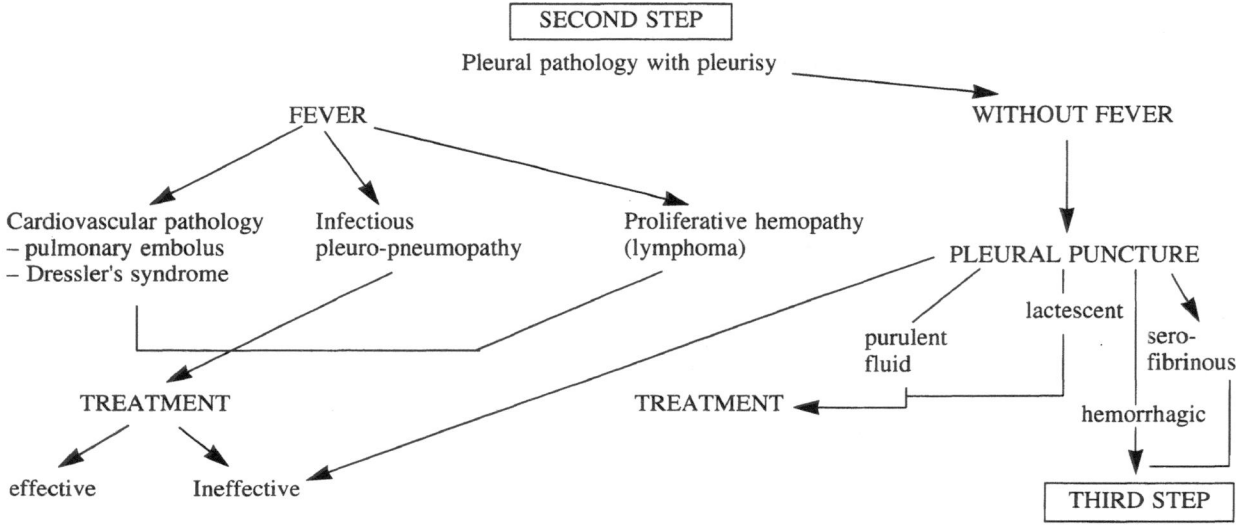

Fig. 34.

3.1. Orientations according to clinical aspects

Pleural effusion may appear in a febrile context with thoracic pain and respiratory difficulty, whose severity is proportional to the intrapleural fluid volume and to the possible compression of mediastinal structures. There are three possible diagnoses:

– pleurisy secondary to a pneumopathy. This may become purulent pleurisy if treatment is delayed [17];

– pleurisy as a complication of a cardiovascular disease such as pulmonary embolus or myocardial infarction. The clinical context must lead to reasses-

sing the diagnosis and to confirmation of undetected pulmonary embolus or Dressler's syndrome [18, 19];

– pleurisy within the framework of a developing lymphoma type of proliferative hemopathy. Pleural effusion develops rapidly and can even become bilateral. Clinical examination and CT-scan may detect adenopathies whose biopsy examinations permit establishment of a diagnosis which necessitates immediate treatment.

These three diagnoses, once made, put an end to pleural investigations. But pleural effusion may develop more insidiously, or recur after treatment of a condition considered initially as infectious in origin. Routine anteroposterior, lateral, and lateral decubitus chest X-ray films permit evaluation of the size of the fluid effusion in the majority of cases.

However there may exist small effusions for which routine radiographic evaluation proves inadequate and here the diagnostic superiority of thoracic ultrasound has been emphasized by several authors [20, 21]. CT-scan allows confirmation of pleurisy in all cases and also provides precise information concerning the lung parenchyma, the pleura, and the mediastinum [22-25].

In the presence of pleural effusion, the occupational and pathologic history, and deficiency conditions associated with the patient, certain diagnoses may be suspected. Thus the previous presence (sometimes several years before) of either a malignant breast or gynecologic tumor in the female, or a pulmonary, renal or ENT tumor in the male, will suggest the possibility of a pleural metastasis. Possible occupational or domestic exposure to asbestos, even of short duration or a long time previously, must suggest consideration of mesothelioma or benign asbestos pathology [26, 27]. Similarly, the history is of great importance when evidence is found of radiotherapy, chemotherapy, or long-term medical treatment. There is abundant literature concerning the direct action of physical or chemical agents on the lymphatic system and the physiologic exchanges of the pleural cavity [28, 29]. Pleurisy can also be due to rheumatoïd arthritis, lupus erythematosis, sarcoidosis, Churg and Strauss syndrome, or Waldenström's disease [30-36]. These various diagnoses suggested by the history and clinical aspects call for confirmation.

3.2. Orientations according to the appearance of the pleural fluid

Pleural aspiration constitutes a decisive step in the diagnostic algorithm [37]. It must be nontraumatic in order not to modify the biochemical characteristics of the fluid obtained [38]. In our department, this is done with patient in supine position, at a point situated on the mid-axillary line when the effusion is free in the pleural cavity, or in front of the pleural sac if the effusion is encysted. The aspect of the fluid is a characteristic of great discriminative value [3]. It permits classification of pleurisies into four groups: purulent, chylous, hemorrhagic or serofibrinous. A purulent aspect immediately points to the diagnosis and necessitates drainage [17, 39] while a milky aspect points towards chylothorax, whose treatment and differential diagnosis from chyloid pleurisy rich in cholesterol are well-known [40-42].

The difficulty in making the diagnosis concerns the other two aspects, since serofibrinous and hemorrhagic pleural effusions may be caused by a multitude of causes; these must be approached by various bacteriologic, biochemical, cytologic and enzymatic examinations.

3.3. Orientations according to bacteriology

In obvious purulent pleurisies bacteriologic tests rarely reveal the causal agent [43] ; empiric and probabilistic antibiotic treatment aborts the infection. In pleurisies with so-called "sero-turbid" fluid, where purulent pleurisy is only suspect, the problem may be difficult if bacteriologic tests are negative.

Some authors advise cytologic examination, including notably leukocyte count and pH level determination in the pleural fluid. A leukocyte count $>10,000/mm^3$ [44] and pH < 7.10 are arguments for probable infection, so the practical attitude is the same as for purulent pleurisies. Search for acid-fast bacilli must be envisaged, especially when the patient is over 70 years of age or if the clinical features suggest possible tuberculosis such as depressed immunity, asthenia, anorexia, recent unexplained weight loss, nocturnal sweating, or possible contagion [45]. A mycologic examination may be requested. *Aspergillus* may be involved, especially in pleural effusion complicating surgical excision for aspergilloma [46-48], or pleural effusion may result from *Torulopsus glabrata* colonisation complicated by an esopleural fistula [49]. Similarly, and according to the clinical context, a parasitologic examination may be requested [50, 51].

3.4. Orientations according to the biochemistry

The literature is full of studies of the biochemical characteristics of serofibrinous or hemorrhagic pleural fluids that suggest diagnoses according to more or less well-defined profiles [52-58]. First, a review of the factors that distinguish a transudate from an exudate is necessary. Three factors seem to be agreed: 1) the pleural protein level, 2) the pleural lactate dehydrogenase concentration with its ratio to serum levels, and 3) the pH level in the pleural fluid. The other characteristics of the pleural fluid are not unanimously accepted concerning their diagnostic value (Fig. 35). A hematocrit greater than 50% would be in favor of malignancy. Glycopleuria, if less than 0.5, would suggest rheumatoïd or infectious pleurisy. A high level of amylase suggests of a lesion below the diaphragm, notably pancreatic [59, 60]. A high level of hyaluronic acid is associated with mesothelioma [61], while a high level of carcinoembryonic antigen is in favor of an adenocarcinomatous origin [62]. The different published studies indicate that some quantitative tests can be of prognostic value [63, 64].

3.5. Orientations according to cytology

Cytologic examination and cell count in pleural fluid obtained by non-traumatic pleural aspiration may point to the diagnosis (Fig. 35). Presence of malignant or suspect cells is very discriminative. The red blood cell, leukocyte and lymphocyte counts must be related to the biochemical characteristics of the pleural fluid in order to improve sensitivity in some cases. Thus a leukocyte count greater than 10,000/mm³, associated with a pH level less than 7.10, a low glycopleuria (40mg/ml) and a lactate dehydrogenase level greater than 1,000 U/l, indicates drainage of an aseptic effusion secondary to a pneumopathy [44]. A percentage of lymphocytes from 90 to 95% in the pleural fluid is highly suggestive of tuberculosis [68, 69]. On the other hand, pleural hypereosinophilia as compared to serum levels is probably associated with a benign pathology [70].

At the end of this investigation the diagnosis of purulent pleurisy and/or chylothorax has been made according to the aspect of the fluid and the bacteriologic, cytologic, and biochemical test results. Furthermore, characterization has been made of the two other categories, namely serofibrinous and hemorrhagic pleural effusion. Their diagnoses, dominated by malignant pathology, overlap. Pleural protein, lactate dehydrogenase and pH levels have helped in identifying effusions of the transudate type. These are attributed to either left cardiac failure, nephrotic syndrome, or cirrhosis according to the clinical picture. For effusions of the exudative type, the diagnostic search must proceed to the use of more invasive procedures.

4. The role of pleural needle-biopsy

Pleural needle-biopsy is a simple technique if certain rules are followed. The presence of a pleural effusion, even if small in quantity, permits guidance of the needle. Localisation must be made either on standard X-ray films or by ultrasound. Local anesthesia helps to obtain patient cooperation. Finally, one must

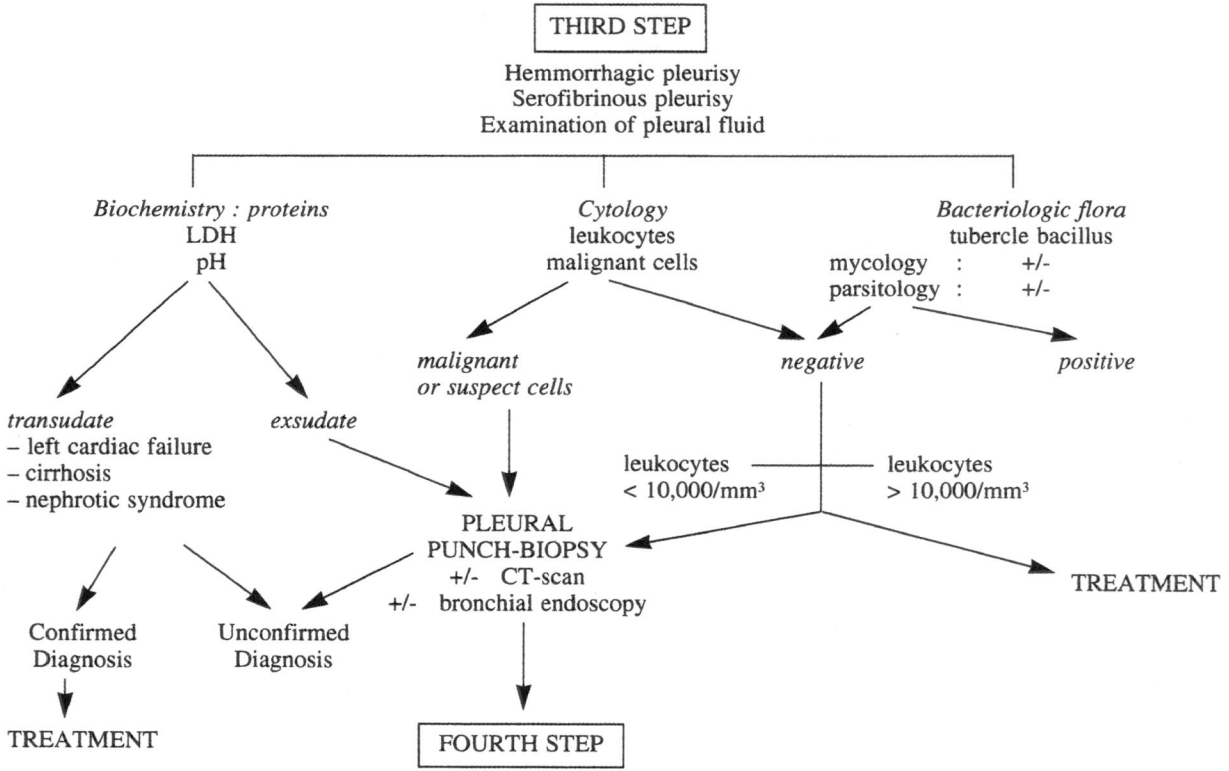

Fig. 35.

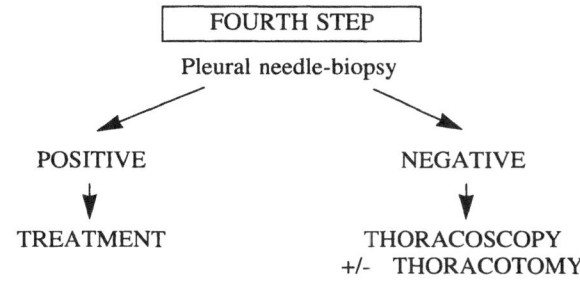

Fig. 36.

be sure that hemostasis is either normal or little affected.

Several types of needles are available, including the Abrams, Cope, or Castellin needles which remain the most classical ones [71-76]. The technique must be rigorous. The tip of the needle, inclined at 45° caudad, must "scrape" the superior edge of the inferior rib of the appropriate intercostal space. Biopsy must produce sufficient material for correct interpretation. Even repeated three times, pleural needle-biopsy yields a poor return. Apart from tuberculosis and diffuse parietal pleural carcinomatosis it is quite difficult and uncertain to obtain specimens from a pathologic area, so much so that a negative pleural needle-biopsy obliges one to consider other diagnostic methods (Fig. 36).

5. The role of thoracoscopy

In the absence of histologic proof, the different diagnoses suggested by the clinical picture and the study of the pleural fluid do not permit initiating treatment. One may be confronted with a more or less abundant serofibrinous or hemorrhagic pleural effusion of the exudate type accompanied by negative pleural needle-biopsy, bacteriologic and cytologic results. On the other hand one may encounter a transudate type of pleural effusion for which the clinical diagnosis and treatment are not conclusive. Lastly, a tumoral pleural pathology may be involved, unaccompanied by pleural effusion, transparietal puncture is either contraindicated or negative. In all cases endoscopic exploration of the pleura is necessary.

Our technique differs little from that described by the majority of authors. Most often two openings are used. The patient is laid on the side opposite to the affected pleura. Neuroleptanalgesia is preferred over local anesthesia for better patient comfort and good exploration of the pleural cavity.

The equipment includes three cold light rigid thoracoscopes (direct, oblique, and lateral vision). These are supplemented by a video camera which permits recording of endoscopic aspects and diagnostic discussion by the operating team. Exploration must be complete. In order to accomplish this, any pleural adhesion encountered must be disrupted with the help of the coagulation forceps. Nodular, mamillated or thickened aspects are in favor of malignancy. A diffuse micronodular aspect may suggest tuberculosis. But even if it seems at the end of an exploration that a pleural carcinosis or a non-specific inflammatory lesion is involved, the final histologic diagnosis is the function of the pathologist to whom large fragments of costal, diaphragmatic parietal pleura and visceral pleura are furnished. Non-specific inflammatory aspects may correspond to pleural effusions associated with malignant tumoral diseases or due to various medical, physical or chemical treatments. These effusions are named as "paraneoplastic" by some authors. Thoracoscopy permits establishment of a sure diagnosis in more than 95% of cases. Apart from this important role in confirming the diagnosis, thoracoscopy can exclude pleural carcinosis when a satellite pleural effusion of a pulmonary tumor is present and thus indicate that excision is still feasible.

6. The role of thoracotomy

There are, however, some cases in which the diagnostic process leads to open pleural biopsy. All extensive pleural tumors inaccessible to thoracoscopy, because it is impossible to create a pneumothorax fall into this category. There are also the cases where biopsies remain negative despite the multiplicity and good quality of specimens obtained. Lastly, there are the rare cases for which a pleurectomy is decided upon. Nevertheless, diagnostic thoracotomy is exceptional at the present time.

7. Conclusion

With such an algorithm for the diagnostic process, the incidence of unidentified pleurisies should fall below the classical level of 13% reported in the literature [4, 5, 86]. Physiologic and pathophysiologic knowledge permits us to ordinate the various diagnostic methods. It is necessary:

– to rationalise the laboratory tests, avoiding use of a routine series of tests which are sometimes useless and often expensive;

– to determine the correct indications for pleural

aspiration-biopsy while avoiding its use in mechanical pleural effusions whose clinical picture is most often suggestive;

– to expertly perform thoracoscopy and have the least recourse to thoracotomy, which is a traumatic and sometimes useless procedure.

Thus it is clear that a period dominated by laboratory screening is being succeeded by an era profiting from technical progress in thoracoscopy.

References

1. Levallen EC, Carr DT (1955) Pleural effusion: a statistical study of 436 patients. N Engl J Med 252 : 79-83

2. Galy P, Brune J, Dorsit J, Delgrange B, Bernheim J, Lacroze M (1971) Étude statistique de 710 épanchements pleuraux observés dans un service de pneumologie. Lyon Méd 226 : 279-285

3. Boutin C, Viallat J, Pastor J, Pauli AM, Dumoulin B, Barre A (1974) Le diagnostic étiologique des pleurésies. Valeurs des examens biologiques non spécifiques du liquide pleural. Essai de diagnostic automatique. Rev Fr Mal Respir 2 : 151-164

4. Hirsch A, Ruffie P, Nebut M, Bignon J, Chrétien J (1979) Pleural effusion: laboratory tests in 300 cases. Thorax 34 : 106-112

5. Lamy P, Canet B, Martinet Y, Lamaze R (1980) Évaluation des moyens diagnostiques dans les épanchements pleuraux. Poumon Cœur 36 : 83-94

6. Sahn SA (1987) Malignant pleural effusions. Sem Resp Med 9 : 1-98

7. Smyrnos NA, Jederlinic PJ, Irwin RS (1990) Pleural effusion in an asymptomatic patient. Spectrum and frequency of causes and management considerations. Chest 97 : 192-196

8. Barnett R (1970) The Pleura. Thorax 25 : 515-524

9. Staub NC, Wiener-Kronish JP, Albertine KH (1984) Physiology of normal transport through the pleura. Physiology of normal liquid and solute exchange in the pleural space. In: Chrétien J (ed.) The Pleura in Health and Disease. Marcel Dekker, New York

10. Wiener-Kronish JP, Berthiaume Y, Albertine KH (1985) Pleural effusions and pulmonary edema. Clinics Chest Med 6 : 509-519

11. Kerbert A (1986) Pathogenesis of pleurisy, pleural fibrosis and mesothelial proliferation. Thorax 41 : 176-189

12. Wiener-Kronish JP, Mattahay MA (1988) Pleural effusions associated with hydrostatic and increased permeability pulmonary edema. Chest 93 : 852-858

13. Cowin B, Addis BJ (1990) Histopathology of the pleura. Journ 57 : 160-175.

14. Blanchon F, Vetter F, Milleron B, Brocard H (1978) Étude clinique des fibromes de la plèvre. Poumon Cœur 34 : 145-152

15. Briselli M, Mark EJ, Dickersin GR (1981) Solitary fibrous tumors of the pleura: eight new cases and review of 360 cases in the literature. Cancer 47 : 2678-2689

16. Thorner M, Maarek H, Bahi M, Carnot F, Buchet R (1989) Les fibromes pleuraux. Évolution des méthodes diagnostiques et aspects anatomopathologiques actuels: A propos de deux observations. Ann Radiol 32 : 305-311

17. Light RW, Girard WM, Jenkinson SG, George RB (1980) Parapneumonia effusions. Am J Med 69 : 507-511

18. Dressler W (1959) The postmyocardial infarction syndrome ; a report of 44 cases. Arch Intern Med 103 : 28-42

19. Stelzner TJ, King TE, Jr Antony VB, Salin SA (1983) The pleuropulmonary manifestations of the postcardiac injury syndrome. Chest 84 : 383-387

20. Grimimki J, Krakowka P, Lypacerniez G (1976) The diagnosis of pleural effusion by ultrasonic and radiologie techniques. Chest 70 : 33-37

21. Kohan JM, Poe RH, Israel RH, Kennedy JD, Benazzy RB, Knellay MC, Greenblatt DW (1986) Value of Chest Ultrasonography versus Decubitus Roentgenography for thoracentesis. Am Rev Respir Dis 113 : 1124-26

22. Kandelman M, Mattei M, Samet P, Chenot L (1977) Tomodensitométrie de la plèvre. Premiers résultats. Rev Fr Mal Resp 5 : 129-32

23. Robinowitz JG, Efremidis SC, Cohen B, Dan Sol, Efremidis A, Chahinian AP, Teirstein AS (1982) Acomparative study of Mesothelioma and Asbestosis using Computed Tomography and Conventional Chest Radiography. Radiology 144 : 453-60

24. Dongay G, Levade M, Lauque D, Carles P, Bollinelli R (1985) Tomodensitométrie de la pathologie pleuro-pulmonaire de l'amiante. Rev Fr Mal Resp 2 : 31-36

25. Maasilta P, Vehmas T, Kinisaan L, Tammilehto L, Mattson K (1991) Correlations between findings at computed tomography (CT) and at thoracoscopy/thoracotomy/autopsy in pleural mesothelioma. Eur Respir J. 4 : 952-54

26. Selikoff IJ, Churg J, Hammond EC (1965) Relation between exposure to asbestos and mesothelioma. N Engl J Med 272 : 560-65

27. Chailleux E, Rembeaux P, Delajartre AY, Deluneau J (1988) Pathologie pleurale bénigne de l'amiante. Rev Pneumol Clin 44 : 166-80

28. Whitcomb ME, Schwarz M (1971) Pleural effusion complicating intensive mediastinal radiation therapy. Am Rev Respir Dis 103 : 100-07

29. Cooper JA Jr, White DA, Matthay RA (1986) Drug-induced pulmonary disease. Am Rev Respir Dis 133 : 321-40

30. Pauli G, Pasquali JL, Jory A, Kopper Schmitt, Kubler MC, Hauptmann G, Roegei E (1981) Les pleurésies rhumatoïdes inaugurales. Intérêt du dosage du complément dans le liquide pleural. A propos de deux cas. Poumon Cœur 37 : 213-17

31. Faurshou P, Francis D, Feramp P (1985) Thoracoscopic, histological and clinical findings in nine cases of rhumatoid pleural effusion. Thorax 40 : 371-75

32. Purnell DC, Baggenstoss AH, Olsen AM (1955) Pulmonary lesions in disseminated lupus erythemaosus. Ann Intern Med 42 : 619-20

33. Winslow WA, Ploss LN, Lotman B (1958) Pleuritis in systemic Lupus erythematosus : Its importance as an cailly manifestation in diagnosis. Ann Intern Med 49 : 70-88

34. Vital Durand D, Dellinger A, Guerin C, Guerin JC, Lerrat F (1984) Pleural Sarcoidosis : One caue presenting with an eosinophilic effusion. Thorax 39 : 468-69

35. Erzurum SC, Underwood GA, Hamilos DL, Waldron JA (1989) Pleural Effusion in Churg Strauss Syndrome Chest 95 : 1357-59

36. Winterbauer RH, Riggins RCK, Ginesman FA, Bauermeister DE (1974) Pleuropulmonary manifestations of Waldenstrom's macro-globulinemia. Chest 66 : 368-75

37. Collins TR, Sahn SA (1987) Thoracentesis Clinical value, complications, technical problems and patient experience. Chest : 91 : 817-22

38. Light RW (1983) Pleural diseases. Lea & Febiger, Philadelphia

39. Riquet M, Debesse B, Bellamy J (1986) Le traitement des pleurésis purulentes aiguës à germes banals de l'adulte. Sem Hôp Paris 62 : 2987-89

40. Straats BA, Effelson RD, Budahn LL, Dines DE, Prakash UBS, Offord K (1980) The lipoprotein profile of chylous and non chylous pleural effusion. Mayo Clin Proc 55 : 700-704

41. Hillerdal G (1985) Chyliform pleural effusion. Chest 88 : 426-428

42. Hamm H, Brohan V, Bohmer R, Missmahl HP (1987) Cholesterol in pleural effusions. A diagnostic aid. Chest 92 : 296-302

43. Bartlett JG, Thadepalli H, Gorbach SL, Eragold SM (1974) Bacteriology of empyema. Lancet i : 338-340

44. Poe RH, Marin MG, Israel RH, Kallay MC Utility of pleural fluid analysis in predicting tube thoracostomy/decortication in parapneumonia effusions

45. Berger HW, Mejia E (1973) Tuberculous pleurisy. Chest 63 : 88-92

46. Krakowka P, Rowinska E, Halweg H (1970) Infection of the pleura by Aspergillus fumigatus. Thorax 25 : 245-253

47. Pesle G, Triboulet F, Gharbi N, Rojas-Miranda A, Merlier M (1980) A propos de 35 cas d'Aspergillose pleurale. Poumon, Cœur 36 : 7-11

48. Einstein HE (ed) Fungus disease of the lungs. Sem Resp Med 9 : 117-222

49. Pesle GD, Gharbi N, Bourcereau J, Levasseur P, Libert JM, Dartevelle P (1982) Torupolis Glabrata, indicateur chirurgical. Soc Fr Mycol Med 11 : 23-26

50. Barrett-Conner E (1982) Parasitic pulmonary disease. Am Rev Respir Dis 126 : 558-563

51. Minh VD, Engle P, Greenwood JR, Predergast TJ, Salnessk K, St Clair R (1981) Pleural paragonimiasis in a South East Asian Refugee. Am Rev Respir Dis 124 : 186-188

52. Levallen EC, Carr DT (1955) Pleural effusion. A statistical study of 436 patients. N Engl Med 252 : 79-83

53. Carr DT, Power MH (1958) Clinical value of measurements of concentration of protein in pleural fluid. N Engl J Med 259 : 926-927

54. Wroblewski F, Wroblewski R (1958) The technical significance of lactic dehydrogenase activity of serous effusions. Ann Intern Med 48 : 813-822

55. Chandraskhar AJ, Palato A, Dubin A, Levine H (1969) Pleural fluid lactic acid dehydrogenase activity and protein content-value in diagnosis. Arch Intern Med 128 : 48-50

56. Light RW, MacGregor MI, Luchsinger PC, Ball WC (1972) Pleural effusions: the diagnostic separation of transudates and exudates. Ann Intern Med 77 : 507-513

57. Saint-Rémy P, Buret J, Radermecker M (1986) Signification des lacticodehydrogénases des épanchements pleuraux. Rev Pneumol Clin 42 : 74-81

58. Degan DP (1977) Données actuelles sur la biochimie du liquide pleural. Rev Fr Mal Resp 5 : 121-128

59. Kramer MR, Saldana MJ, Cepero RJ, Pitchenik AE (1989) High amylase levels in neoplasm-related pleural effusion. Ann Intern Med 110 : 567-569

60. Girbes PRJ, Postmus PE, Jansen W, Vd Jagt EJ, Kleibeuker JH (1990) Massive pleural effusion due to pancreatic pseudocyst. Thorax 45 : 563-564

61. Chn B, Churg A, Tengblad A, Pearie R, McCaugley WTE (1984) Analysis of hyaluronic acid in the diagnosis of malignant mesothelioma. Cancer 54 : 2195-2199

62. Al Saffar N, Hasleton PS (1990) Vimentin, carcinoembryonic antigen and keratin in the diagnosis of mesothelioma, adenocarcinoma and reactive pleural effusions. Eur Respir J 3 : 997-1001

63. Gottehrer A, Taryle DA, Reed CE, Sahn SA (1991) Pleural fluid analysis in malignant mesothelioma. Chest 100 : 1003-1006

64. Pandero-Rodriguez F, Mejias Lopez J (1989) Low glucose and pH levels in malignant pleural effusions. Am Rev Respir Dis 1398 : 663-667

65. Dines DE, Pierre RV, Franzen SJ (1975) The value of cells in the pleural fluid in the differential diagnosis. Mayo Clin Proc 50 : 571-572

66. Marriquand C, Augusseau S, Marriquand J, Breyton M, Paramelle B (1977) Quelques aperçus sur les méthodes d'étude actuelles de la cytologie pleurale. Rev Fr Mal Resp 5 : 113-120

67. Johnston WW (1985) The malignant pleural effusion. A review of cytopathologic diagnosis of 584 specimens from 472 consecutive patients. Cancer 56 : 905-909

68. Light RW, Erozan YS, Ball WC Jr (1973) Cells in pleural fluid: their value in differential diagnosis. Arch Intern Med 132 : 854-860

69. Yam LT (1967) Diagnostic significance of lymphocytes in pleural effusions. Ann Intern Med 66 : 972-982

70. Adelman M, Albelda SM, Gottlied J, Haponik EF (1984) Diagnostic utility of pleural fluid eosinophilia. Am J Med 77 : 915-920

71. Scharer L, Mc Clemant JH (1968) Isolation of tubercle bacilliform needle biopsy specimens of parietal pleura. Am Rev Respir Dis 97 : 466-468

72. Salyer WR, Eggleston JC, Erozan YS (1975) Efficacy of pleural needle biopsy and pleural fluid cytopathology in the diagnosis of malignant neoplasm involving the pleura. Chest 67 : 536-539

73. Migueres J, Jover A, Bouissou H, Rumeau JL, Armisen A, Escamilla R (1981) Place de la ponction-biopsie à l'aiguille et du cytodiagnostic dans le diagnostic des pleurésies malignes. Poumon-Cœur 37 : 29-34

74. Poe RH, Israel RH, Utell MJ, Hell WJ et al (1984) Sensitivity, specificity and predictive values of closed pleural biopsy. Arch Intern Med 144 : 325-328

75. Morrone N, Algranti E, Barreto E (1987) Pleural biopsy with Cope and Abrams Needles. Chest 92 : 1050-1052

76. Ogirala RG, Agarwa V, Alorich TK (1989) Raja pleural biopsy needle. A comparison with the Abrams needle in experimental pleural effusion. Am Rev Respir Dis 139 : 984-987

77. Boutin C, Cargnino P, Viallat JR (1981) Thoracoscopy in malignant effusion. Am Rev Respir Dis 124 : 588-592

78. Boutin C, Viallat JR, Cargnino P, Farisse P, Choux R (1981) La thoracoscopie en 1980. Revue Générale Poumon-Cœur 37 : 11-19

79. Boutin C, Viallat JR, Cargnino P, Farisse P, Irisson M, Rey F, Velardocchio JM (1985) Thoracoscopy: In Chrétien J (ed) The pleura in health and disease. Marcel Dekker, New York : 587-622

80. Hucker J, Bhatnager NK, Al Jilaihawi AN, Forester-Wood CP (1991) Thoracoscopy in the diagnosis and management of recurrent pleural effusions. Ann Thorac Surg 52 : 1145-1147

81. Corrin B, Addis BJ (1990) Histopathology of the pleura. Respiration 57 : 160-175

82. Swierenga J, Wagenaar JP, Bergstein P (1974) The value of thoracoscopy in the diagnosis and treatment of diseases affecting the pleura and lung. Pneumologie 151 : 11-18

83. Canto A, Blasco E, Casillas M, Zarza AG, Perdilla J, Pastor J, Tarazona V, Paris F (1977) Thoracoscopy in the diagnosis of pleural effusion. Thorax 32 : 550-554

84. Boutin C, Carcnino P, Viallat JR, Scarbonchi Efimieff T (1979) La thoracoscopie dans les cancers métastatiques de la plèvre. Rev Fr Mal Respir 7 : 625-627

85. Wihlm JM (1990) La place de la pleuroscopie dans le bilan pré-opératoire du cancer bronchique. Ann Chir Thorac Cardio-vasc 44 : 139-142

86. Chrétien J, Maillard JM, Brouet G (1970) Épanchements pleuraux d'évolution chronique et d'étiologie indéterminée : pleurésies chroniques aspécifiques. J Fr Med Chir Thor 24 : 271

The role of thoracoscopy in the treatment of chronic pleural effusion

P. Baldeyrou

1. Introduction

Chronic pleural effusion is defined as an effusion which persists longer than 2 or 3 weeks with negative diagnostic test results. This definition is expanded to include the range of pleural effusions with or without a diagnosis that persist longer than this period. Two problems must be resolved in these effusions, namely those of making the diagnosis and prescribing treatment, since pleurisy constitutes an autonomous pathologic entity.

Persistance of diagnostic uncertainty complicates therapeutic management, in that the necessity of thoracoscopy for making the diagnosis often also leads to its use for endopleural treatment. Cancer as an etiology is of greatest importance.

Both the general condition and the prognosis are taken into account in selection of treatment in order not to burden unnecessarily patients who are for the most part in the preterminal stage of disease.

Treatment includes evacuative aspiration and drainage associated with intrapleural injections, talc pleurodesis using thoracoscopy, and rarely pleuroperitoneal shunts or thoracotomy.

2. Etiology

The first ranking cause of chronic pleural effusion is cancer. Foremost is primary bronchopulmonary cancer but secondary tumors are also quite often found. Among the latter, breast cancer is the most frequent source.

About 40% of tumoral pleurisies are caused by adenocarcinomas of unknown origin.

Mesotheliomas are responsible for 10% of malignant pleurisies [8]. They are characterized by direct invasion of adjacent tissues, especially the thoracic wall, and in particular the sites of biopsies and drainage. Therefore, systematic radiotherapy focussed on the routes of biopsy and thoracoscopy is justified according to Boutin [2] and Guérin [3] in cases of mesothelioma.

Next in frequency after chronic pleurisy of tumoral origin come those which stem from a heart problem, especially venous pulmonary hypertension. Global treatment of the cause is indicated in these cases; however, self-regenerating pleurisy may require local treatment.

The same autonomy of effusion is found in ascitic hydrothorax caused by increased abdominal pressure that activates pleuroperitoneal exchanges. Cure of this particular type of pleurisy can increase the ascites, so careful selection of treatment is indicated.

Many causes are responsible for other chronic pleurisies, including general diseases such as chylothorax or lymphoma. The chronicity of a pleural effusion suggests resorting to pleurodesis.

3. Methods of treatment

Beside repetitive evacuative aspiration according to need, which is reserved either for patients in very precarious preterminal stage disease or for those with an assumed transitory condition, two therapeutic procedures are preferentially employed.

These are as follows:
1) talc pleurodesis under thoracoscopy,
2) puncture and/or drainage with injections of

drugs. Indications are very limited for the Denver pleuroperitoneal shunt and open thorax surgery.

Prior to treatment selection, verification of the free condition of the pleural cavity is made either through films with the patient in lateral decubitus on the effusion side or through ultrasound. The latter verifies the mobility of the pleural effusion. When effusion volume is significant, total or subtotal evacuation is necessary in order to permit reexpansion of the pulmonary parenchyma filling the pleural cavity and refilling the thoracic cavity.

3.1. Thoracoscopic talc pleurodesis

Among the 90 thoracoscopies personally performed, 64 were for talc pleurodesis of a tumoral pleurisy. Thoracoscopic talc pleurodesis is done under local or general anesthesia according to availabilities and schools. We prefer general anesthesia which seems to us to be easier, faster and less painful. Thoracoscopy is carried out with introduction of one or two trocar(s) into the 5th or 6th intercostal space on each side of the middle axillary line. Areas of partial adhesion are freed. Talc is dusted onto the parietal pleura under visual control so that it is regularly distributed. We use about 5 ml of talc [3], i.e. 1 or 2 bottles of pressurized talc.

Absence of pathologic diagnosis in pleurisy favors using thoracoscopy since it permits simultaneous determination of the diagnosis by peroperative pathologic examination as well as performance of symptomatic treatment by pleurodesis.

Suction drainage is started using one or two drains which we prefer to be of small caliber (18 F) and multiperforated. Drains are only withdrawn when there is no more drainage or at the latest on the 8-10th day following operation (average 2.7 days) [1].

Thoracoscopic talc pleurodesis yields from 87% [1] to 90% [3] of good results. Failures occur when the lung is incarcerated by the effusion or shrunken by a thick neoplastic visceral pleura, leading to mediocre or insufficient reexpansion.

Global mortality is around 1% [9]. But in fact exact assessment of complications is very difficult since talc pleurodesis is performed most often in a palliative context. All of the severe or lethal complications in the treatment register for chronic pleural effusion have arisen in this context [1]. Air embolism is exceptional, fever is not unusual and temporary, and pleural iatrogenic infection is rare since it is prevented by prophylactic antistaphylococcic antibiotic treatment on one hand and by postoperative drainage on the other [4].

Local complications include neoplastic seeding along the puncture pathway, especially in cases of mesothelioma, occasional subcutaneous crepitations (always benign), and occasional parietal infections.

3.2. Intrapleural injections

Drugs, injected either directly or through a drain, and repetitive aspiration were for a long time the only treatment proposed for chronic pleurisy. Then intrapleural injections following evacuation were introduced. The value of this technique is still debatable for many physicians since the results are very difficult to evaluate; the success rate is probably overall less than 50%. Pneumologists and surgeons more willingly use drainage. We prefer drainage to totally evacuate effusions with a small latex drain (14 F) before drug injection. Using this method we have performed a hundred pleurodesis without a single complication, only in patients whose condition precluded talc pleurodesis. If the parenchymal reexpansion is complete or almost complete, the operation is carried out under the same conditions as for thoracoscopy with intrapleural injection then clamping the drain for 48 hours. This technique may be performed without difficulty even if prior partial adhesion exists and it may be repeated. After injection, for a better distributing of the drug over the pleural surface, the patient is mobilized for 5 minutes into each of the following positions: dorsal, ventral, right and left lateral decubitus; sloping; and standing. After 48 hours the drain is resuctioned for a few hours then withdrawn. This technique has no complications apart from fever of about 38°C lasting 24 - 48 hours.

Either tetracycline diluted in 100 ml physiologic saline or antimitotics are the drugs injected. Results reported for tetracycline are quite variable in the literature with as much as 80% good results [10]. However good technical conditions are never totally obtained including effusion evacuation by drainage, good drug dispersion, and subsequent reaspiration. Nonetheless tetracycline is undoubtably responsable for more late recurrences than antimitotics. Bleomycin is the most effective with 80% good results reported [7]; we inject 100 mg bleomycin diluted in 100 ml physiologic saline. Nevertheless, rapid pleural reabsorption of bleomycine occurs and its general toxicity is compounded with that of other antimitotics already administer to the patient. Therefore, for us the choice between tetracycline and bleomycin depends essentially on the increased toxicity bleomycin may produce in patients treated for cancer.

3.3. Other techniques

The Denver pleuroperitoneal drainage method is

attractive but not yet in general use. The major objection to this technique is the necessity for the patient himself or a person in his immediate surroundings to make the subcutaneous pump work, which implies both personal commitment and adequate physical condition. In our experience these two requirements are rarely met. In fact, this only method was indicated in 4% of the 358 chronic pleural effusion cases treated by Ponn et al [6].

Thoracotomy is a severe operation whose aim is to carry out parietal pleurectomy with parenchymal decortication. It is burdened with a mortality at from 5% to 10% and a considerable morbidity, including hemorrhagic or septic complications and painful sequelae. Thus, it can only be an exceptional indication reserved for still young patients in good general health, who have no pleuropulmonary adhesions but whose lung is totally incarcerated, and contracted on its pedicle. It may also be indicated in cases of complete failure of intrapleural techniques [9].Adequate results were obtained in 90% of surgical cases reported by Martini [5] despite 2 to 4 weeks' hospitalization.

4. Indications

The following three aspects must be considered prior to embarking on a treatment modality:
– the etiologic diagnosis has been made or on the contrary remains in doubt;
– whether or not the general health and overall prognosis point to prolonged survival;
– whether or not the pulmonary parenchyma reexpands.

Absence of an etiologic diagnosis suggests diagnostic thoracoscopy, which also permits talc pleurodesis, but only if the lung parenchyma reoccupies its normal place after evacuation of fluid.

When the general condition is mediocre and life expectancy reduced to a matter of weeks, the reasonable choice is simple drainage with injection of either tetracyline or bleomycin. When pleural adhesion is already partially present, as demonstrated in the lateral decubitus films, chemical pleurodesis via the drain is the method of choice. The choice between antibiotics or antimitotics is linked to the toxicity of the latter which varies according to their previous administration to the patient. In this situation, relatively incomplete reexpansion of the parenchyma leaving small air pockets does not contraindicate an endopleural injection since the resultant pleurodesis will most often be adequate enough to avoid any future necessity for aspiraton. On the contrary, gene-

ral corticosteroid administration at doses higher than 20 mg/day of prednisone, for instance, should be decreased significantly from 15 to 20 days before intrapleural operation and for at least the same amount of time afterwards since in our experience, attempts at pleurodesis seem to be highly negatively influenced by corticosteroid therapy.

In all other cases thoracoscopic talc pleurodesis is the treatment of choice for chronic pleural effusion, with the same reservations as in injection of drugs regarding temporary decrease of corticosteroid levels.

Exceptional situations remain to be discussed:
– major hydropneumothorax without any pleural adhesion, in which decortication with pleurectomy may be considered according to the overall prognosis;
– major pleural fluid production (up to 1 liter or more per day) in relation to a tumoral process. If thoracoscopy or an operation has been performed, prenature withdrawal of drains must be avoided (i.e. not before 10 days postoperatively), and reliable efficacity of cytostatic drugs in stabilizing disease is called for. It is probably in these very limited indications that the Denver shunt device finds its usefulness since it does not aim to evacuate the effusion completely but only to decrease dyspnea [6, 7].

5. Conclusion

Chronic pleural effusion is treated by 2 types of local techniques including thoracoscopic talc pleurodesis and chemical pleurodesis. The treatment of choice is talc pleurodesis since it is more effective. Moreover, it can be performed electively when a patient needs thoracoscopic diagnosis. Chemical pleurodesis is somewhat less effective but much more tolerable in very compromised patients.

References

1. Aelony Y, King R, Boutin C (1991) Thoracoscopic talc poudrage for chronic recurrent pleural effusion. Ann Int Med 115 : 778-782
2. Boutin C, Rey F, Viallat JR (1986) Étude randomisée de l'efficacité du talcage par thoracoscopie et de l'instillation de tétracyclines dans le traitement des pleurésies cancéreuses récidivantes. Rev Mal Resp 2 : 2374-2380
3. Guerin JC (1992) Place de la thorascocopie dans le diagnostic et le traitement des épanchements pleuraux. Premières journées d'Endoscopie Thoracique Thérapeutique, Paris, France, 24-25 janvier 1992
4. Macalpine LG, Hulks G, Thomson NC (1990) Manage-

ment of recurrent malignant pleural effusion in the United Kingdom. Thorax 45 : 699-701

5. Martini N, Bains MS, Beattie EJ (1975) Indications for pleurectomy in malignant effusion. Cancer 35 : 734-738

6. Ponn RB, Blancafor RJ, D'Agostino RS, Kierman ME, Toole AL, Stern H. (1991) Pleuro-peritoneal shunting for intractable pleural effusions. Ann Thorac Surg 51 : 605-609

7. Ostrowski MJ (1986) An assessment of the long term results of controlling the reaccumulation of malignant

effusion using intra cavitory Bleomycin. Cancer 57 : 721-727

8. Sahn SA (1988) The Pleura. Am Rev Respir Dis 138 : 184-234

9. Wakabayashi A (1991) Expanded applications of diagnostic and therapeutic thoracoscopy. J Thorac Cardio Vasc Surg 102 : 721-723

10. Zacoznik A, Oswald SG, Languib NM (1992) Intrapleural Tetracycline in malignant pleural effusion. A randomised Study. Cancer 51 : 752-755

Principles of the thoracoscopic approach

A. Wakabayashi

1. General considerations

Blebs or emphysematous bullae do not have mucosal linings and are not true cysts, but contain air. Therefore they are pseudopneumocysts (PPCs) of the lungs. Many of PPCs do not cause any harm and are often found incidentally at autopsy. It is not entirely clear how they are formed and in this chapter, the pathogenesis will not be discussed. When PPCs rupture (spontaneous pneumothorax) the air escapes into the pleural space, causing dyspnea. When PPCs take up a significant amount of the intrapleural space, the patients develop dyspnea (diffuse bullous emphysema). In this chapter, thoracoscopic treatment of these two clinical manifestations of PPCs will be discussed.

Spontaneous pneumothorax is a common problem and much discussed in the literature. The appropriate treatment plan should be based on an understanding of the underlying cause, which is usually related to the patient's age. Although spontaneous pneumothorax can occur in any age group, it is more prevalent among the young. Less commonly, it occurs in elderly patients with severe chronic obstructive pulmonary disease (COPD), which presents an extremely difficult challenge to the surgeon. Diffuse bullous emphysema is a chronic debilitating disease among elderly smokers or ex-smokers with COPD. The bullae are diffusely distributed, involving both sides of the lungs and all lobes, defying satisfactory surgical removal. Until homologous lung transplantation became practical, there was no definitive treatment for diffuse bullous emphysema available.

The original thoracoscope was developed in 1915 by Jacobaeus [1] to facilitate the artificial pneumothorax in the treatment of cavernous tuberculosis. The device consisted or a metal hollow tube with a small light bulb at its tip, which is alike a Jacksonian pediatric bronchoscope, and a soldering gun type probe which was used for cauterization. The thoracoscope was utilized in the treatment of spontaneous pneumothorax by a few investigators. Waterman [2] reported the first application of the original Jacobaeus' thorascoscope in a young woman with ruptured bleb in 1950. Ratliff et al [3] reported a case with spontaneous hemopneumothorax in 1977. They used a flexible bronchoscope as a thoracoscope and cauterized the apical bleeder with a brush biopsy forceps. In 1978, Takeno [4] reported the use of liquid glue sprayed over the ruptured bleb under a thoracoscopic control. In 1989, Wakabayashi [5] reported the initial group of patients with spontaneous pneumothorax treated with thoracoscope and electrocautery. A high failure rate was encountered due to mostly inappropriate instrumentation. In an attempt to improve the result, carbon dioxide (CO_2) laser was adopted to ablate blebs or bullae. The preliminary results were reported in 1990 [6]. In these studies, the thoracoscope was used to identify the underlying lesions and to stop air leaks or to ablate the blebs or emphysematous bullae under direct vision. In contrast to these direct approaches, the thoracoscope has been used by many investigators to determine the mode of therapy for spontaneous pneumothorax [7, 8]. If the underlying cause is found to be emphysematous bullae, the patients are treated by open thoracotomy and lung resection. If blebs are found then sclerosing procedure (pleurodesis) is carried out using talc powder [9], tetracycline [8] or neodymium yttrium aluminum garnet (Nd: YAG) laser [10] under thoracoscopic control.

Thoracoscopic laser treatment of diffuse bullous emphysema was first performed in May of 1989

[11]. Since then, more than 80 patients were treated successfully by this new technique. This procedure has expanded the application of laser thoracoscopy and produced significant improvements both subjectively and objectively in the majority of patients. This is an example that the thoracoscopy is used not only as an alternative to thoracotomy but also has opened a new horizon in creating a new treatment.

2. Classification of pseudopneumocysts of the lungs (Table 1)

In order to understand the thoracoscopic treatment of PPCs it is necessary to describe the classification, based on the thoracoscopic findings. PPCs of the lungs are traditionally classified mainly on the histology. Additional information such as X-ray findings and pulmonary function are also considered [12-13]. However, the traditional classification has little practical value in determining the mode of treatment and I therefore proposed a new classification based on the thoracoscopic findings [5]. This has proved very useful in planning the mode of thoracoscopic treatment. Blebs are defined as the same way as in the traditional classification. They are small subpleural air cysts of less than 10 mm in diameter, with very thin walls which have no blood-vessels. They are commonly found in the apical area of the upper lobes but also frequently along the margins of the upper and lower lobes. Blebs are the most common cause of spontaneous pneumothorax among young patients, rupture being commonly seen between the age 17 and 29 years. Bullae are classified into three types. Type I bullae have a single lumen without trabeculae. They are medium to large in size and have thick walls with abundant blood-vessels. A few bronchial communications are present which act as one-way valves. Large type I bullae are readily recognizable on plain chest films. For evaluating patients with COPD for thoracocopic laser treatment, we routinely obtain computed tomography (CT) of the lungs without contrast. In order to study the dynamic aspects of diffuse bullous emphysema, we have been using a fast scanner CT video (Imatron). It was interesting to observe that their sizes remain unchanged during respiration. Frequently a pendulum motion of a large bulla compressing the main bronchus is observed during expiration. On rare occasions, the air moves in and out of the type I bullae, which are referred to as ventilating bullae. Since they do not have any capillaries for gas exchange, they simply act as a dead space. The internal surface of type I bullae is characteristically smooth and no trabeculae exist. When they reach an enormous size, they cause

Table 1. Classification of pseudopneumocysts (PPCs) of the lungs

Blebs :	Subpleural PPCs, less than 1 cm in diameter
Bullae :	Intraparenchymal PPCs, larger than 1 cm in diameter
I	Single lumen, medium to large, a few communication with bronchial systems
II	Conglomerate of small to medium bullae, most commonly confined to apex
III	Medium to large, filled with trabeculae, numerous communications with bronchialsystems

dyspnea. Traditionally, type I bullae are the ideal indication for surgical bullectomy. In general, however, it is rare to find only a single type I bulla and commonly it is mixed with type III bullae. Type II bullae are a conglomerate of small to medium intraparenchymal bullae. They are usually confined to the apex of the lungs. Each bulla has a smooth internal surface. When they are opened, numerous septi separating individual bullae are found. They are found in any age group. Type II bullae are the second most common but the most common cause of spontaneous pneumothorax that requires surgical intervention. Ruptured type II bullae are seen among slightly older patients than ruptured blebs, aged 22 to 40 years. Characteristically, they are clearly demarcated from the normal lung parenchyma, so that surgical excision provides an excellent result. Type III are intraparenchymal bullae, diffusely distributed in all three lobes and containing numerous trabeculae. They are the most common cause of diffuse bullous emphysema causing dyspnea. Traditionally, surgical excision of type III bullae has had a high mortality with poor functional results because of the absence of demarcation between the normal lung and the bullae. Various stages of maturity of type III bullae are observed. Early stages are characterized by diffuse and very small intraparenchymal bullae intermingled with functioning lung parenchyma. The most mature form mimics type I bullae and is called pseudo-type I, being frequently indistinguishable from true type I bullae on CT films. Their appearance at thoracospopy is also very similar to that of type I. However, when they are opened, residual trabeculae are always found, usually at their bases. They are also good candidates for traditional surgical bullectomy. The majority of patients with diffuse bullous emphysema have a mixture of type III bullae of different stages.

In planning the thoracoscopic treatment of PPCs of the lungs, preoperative assessment ot the types of PPCs is very useful. PPCs become surgical problems when they rupture, causing spontaneous pneumothorax or dyspnea.

3. Treatment planning for PPC of the lungs

3.1. Spontaneous pneumothorax

Blebs are not identifiable on either plain or CT films. It is impossible to detect type II bullae on a plain chest film, though they can sometimes be identified on CT films as small bubble-like cysts. Type I bullae are frequently seen as a large air-pocket on a plain chest film. Type III bullae cannot be identified on plain chest films, except mature forms of pseudotype I. The only radiographic evidence of type III bullae is hyperinflation of the lungs, increased anterior-posterior diameter of the chest and flattened diaphragm. In some patients, local bulging of the chest wall indicates the presence of underlying bullae. Type III bullae are more easily demonstrated on CT films.

The cause of spontaneous pneumothorax is usually unclear until surgery, except for patients with a known history of COPD. The most common cause of spontaneous pneumothorax among young, otherwise healthy males is ruptured blebs. However, a significant number have ruptured type II bullae which require different treatment techniques. Therefore, in treating young patients with spontaneous pneumothorax, one must be prepared for type II bullae. If ruptured blebs are found instead they can be effectively ablated by electrocautery. If ruptured type II bullae are found, the CO_2 or Nd: YAG contact laser is turned on, which takes only a couple of minutes. The laser equipment should be available in the operating room when patients with spontaneous pneumothorax are treated by thoracoscopy. Endoloop, 4-0 PDSII suture with an SH needle, and an Endo-GIA 30 stapler are also kept in the operating room.

The patients with ruptured type III bullae (COPD patients) require careful evaluation. In addition to plain chest films, CT films of the chest should be obtained. They are, in general, elderly and chronic smokers or ex-smokers and ischemic heart disease is fairly common. Right heart failure is also not uncommon. Supraventricular arhythmias are also a common finding. Preoperative EKG is routinely obtained. In contrast to an elective operation for diffuse bullous emphysema, surgical intervention to ruptured type III bullae is a medical emergency. Therefore, we do not subject these patients to any further investigation for coronary artery disease, e.g. coronary arteriography. Flow-velocity spirometry is inaccurate in the presence of massive air leaks, so that pulmonary function study is not made. Arterial blood gases, electrolytes, creatinine and BUN are checked. The patients will probably require prolonged postoperative ventilatory support and the duration of tube thoracostomy is long. Therefore, they will require an indwelling arterial line and Swan-Ganz catheter placement perioperatively. The chosen laser equipment is prepared. In addition, a surgical tray for conventional thoracotomy should be available in the operating room.

3.2. Diffuse bullous emphysema

Indications and patient selection for laser bullectomy will be discussed later. In contrast to ruptured type III bullae causing spontaneous pneumothorax, the treatment is purely elective and the patient should be thoroughly screened. The surgical treatment of diffuse bullous emphysema is extremely demanding and requires as much effort as a lung transplantation team. The team should include pneumologists, radiologists, anesthesiologists, infectious disease specialists, cardiologists, operating room personnel, respiration therapists, intensive care nurses, medical floor nurses, physical therapists, occupational therapists and nutritionists. The majority of patients come from out of town. Their hospital stay is long, and even after discharge they have to stay near the hospital for at least 10 days to two weeks. This creates a substantial socioeconomic burden on the patients and their families. Therefore, social workers and clinical psychologists are frequently involved in patient care. The organization of the team is, however, not as extensive as that for lung transplantation. If this type of team cannot be organized, elective treatment of diffuse bullous emphysema should not be attempted.

Since most patients with diffuse bullous emphysema are elderly chronic or ex-smokers, the incidence of significant occlusive coronary artery disease is high. We have been evaluating the value of Imatron screening of calcium deposits in the coronary arteries. If a significant amount of calcium is found in the left main coronary artery or proximal triple vessels, the patients are subjected to selective coronary angiography. So far, this highly sensitive test has not given positive results; a false-positive test is too common. If there is any suspicion of occult occlusive coronary artery disease, we obtain a dobutamine echocardiogram since these patients cannot be stressed on a treadmill long enough to disclose the coronary disease. If the evidence suggests that they may have a significant occlusive disease, the patient must have a coronary arteriography.

4. Equipment

4.1. Optic/video systems and instruments

The brightness and optic resolution of the optic/video systems are two essential components of successful thoracoscopy. The most advanced optic/video systems offered by several companies are all similar and satisfactory. A xenon light source (OLV-U20) with automatic exposure control is used, the old halogen light source being dark and unsatisfactory. The automatic iris offered by Olympus is a very important feature which prevents annoying glare.

Some video cameras give too much magnification and are difficult to use. Mistakes can be made with these cameras because of failure to identify what is being seen. The Olympus video camera system (OTV-S2) with a direct coupler is very satisfactory. The screw-on direct coupler is favored over a conventional clip-on type video camera; not only does it improve optic resolution but it also makes rotation of the angled thoracoscope much easier. A videotape recorder and optional hard copy printer (Sony mavigraph color video printer) are routinely used. The quality of color prints is suboptimal but should be adequate for documentation. I use a 19 inch color monitor as a primary monitor and a 13 inch color monitor as a second monitor. These two monitors are connected with a cable and housed inside a mobile cart (Cart-4). It is very important that the monitors be mobile since they must be moved up and down all the time during the procedure.

Use of the Olympus rigid thoracoscopes exclusively for the past two years has shown them to be very satisfactory. A screw-on video camera is preferred. A 30° scope is used in about 70 % of the time and found to be very versatile. For spontaneous pneumothorax, for instance, I use the 30° thoracoscope throughout the procedure. In brief, the 30° degree thorascoscope is used for the initial inspection. If the target is straight down towards the mediastinum, then the thoracoscope is changed for a 0° degree instrument, which not only makes orientation easier but offers better optical resolution and brightness than an angled instrument. A flexible fiberoptic thoracoscope (9 mm) is now commercially available, whose brightness and resolution are approximately 90 % of those of the rigid scopes. Its advantage is that it has no blind angle. Since it can visualise the entire intrapleural space without being pressed hard against the intercostal nerve, postoperative pain is less than with the use of the rigid thoracoscope. It is frustrating and very time-consuming to clean the lens of the thoracoscope frequently. An air/fluid flushing mechanism is essential, especially for the flexible thoracoscope, since it is technically more difficult to pull this out of the trocar than a rigid thoracoscope. However, the air/fluid flushing mechanism of the current model is suboptimal and needs to be improved.

Curved instruments are essential in thoracoscopy. Table 2 lists reusable operating instruments required

Table 2. Reusable Operating Instruments (Olympus) required for thoracoscopie treatment of PPCs

Trocar, 10 and 5 mm
Grasping forceps, 5 mm, straight, left and right curved
Spatula/cautery, malleable, 5 mm
Hoock scissors, 5 mm, straight, left and right curved
Needle catcher, 5 mm
Introducer, 5 mm
Knot pusher, 5 mm
Shark sucker, 10 mm, straight and curved

for thoracoscopic treatment of spontaneous pneumothorax. Disposable instruments are expensive and whenever possible reusable instruments should be used. However, disposable instruments should always be available in the operating room as a back-up. Also, hook scissors tend to get dull very quickly and nothing is more frustrating. Disposable hook scissors are much sharper than reusable scissors and should be available as a back-up. Reusable spatula, needle holder, and grasper are superior to disposable instruments.

4.2. Lasers

4.2.1. Carbon Dioxide Laser

The carbon dioxide (CO_2) laser (Fig. 37) is one of the oldest surgical laser equipments and least expensive. Since its beams are invisible, it is combined with a low-energy red, helium-neon laser. The CO_2 laser is delivered through a series of hollow metal tubes containing reflecting mirrors. This articulated arm has a counterbalance but is frequently clumsy to move around. The alignment of the laser equipment must be periodically checked by the engineer. The CO_2 laser is used in thoracoscopy not only for cutting the tissues but also for shrinking PPCs. Since the CO_2 laser is absorbed by water in living tissues, it is an excellent cutter. However, it is less effective in coagulating blood than an argon or neodymium-yttrium-aluminum-garnet (Nd: YAG) laser. For cutting purposes, the maximal output of 40 watts is sufficient. Another very useful function of the CO_2 laser is to shrink PPCS of the lungs and weld the lung parenchyma. For these indications, a low energy level of the CO_2 laser of less than 6 watts, is used. Since the tissue penetration of the CO_2 laser is less than 100 μ at this energy level, this is the safest laser for use with a thorascoscope. Even if the laser beam inadvertently hits the pulmonary artery or aorta, the adventitia only shrinks a little and there is no risk of perforation. The laser beams are delivered via either

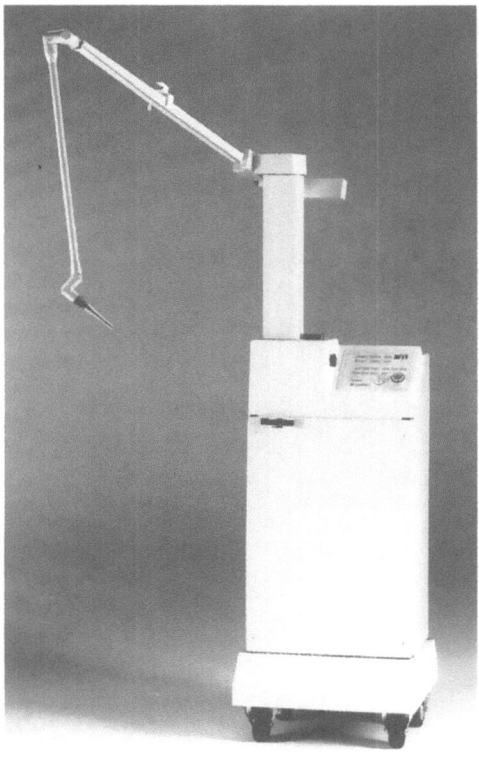

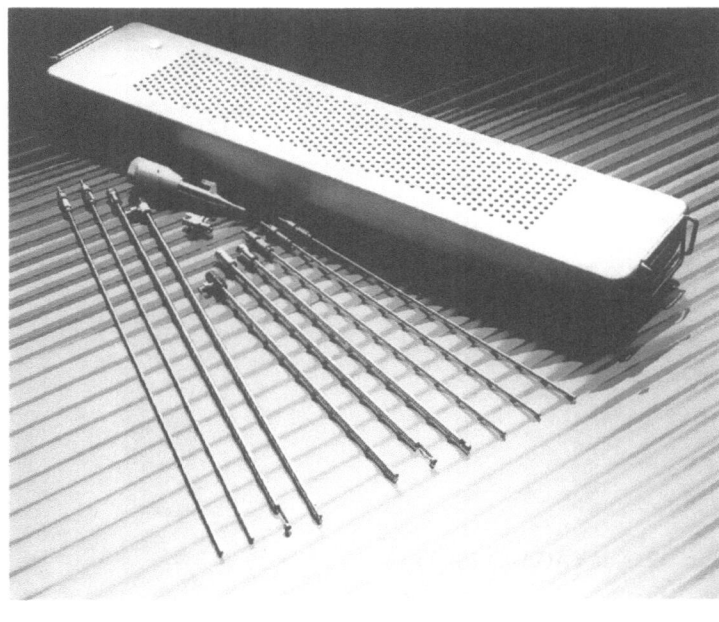

38

Fig. 37. CO$_2$ laser Unit (Coherent)

Fig. 38. Waveguide (Coherent)

a laserscope (Olympus) or a waveguide™ (Fig. 38) (Coherent, Palo Alto, CA). The laserscope is used with a Gallerian focusing device. In order to deliver a very low-power density, the beams are maximally defocussed by this device prior to use. This will reduce the risk of perforation of a PPC. Since the CO$_2$ laser beams are delivered through the thoracoscope, it is easier to administer the laser through the laserscope than through the waveguide™. The disadvantage of the laserscope is that the junction tends to become loose and lose alignment easily, especially when the laserscope is moved around in a wide range. In contrast, the wageguide has a fixed focus and the spot size of the laser beams is adjusted by the distance between its tip and the target. Also it requires a second trocar for insertion. However, it is very stable and can be used from any direction without losing alignment. The gooling CO$_2$ gas of the waveguide™ also disperses the laser fumes. The waveguide™ has different attachment for different applications. For instance, a back-stop probe is used to divide the fibrous adhesions. A metal back-stop prevents injury of the tissues behind the adhesions. The Shark sucker is connected to a smoke evacuator and retained in the chest cavity. Weak continuous suction is maintained to evacuate laser

smoke. If strong suction is applied, the tissues are sucked against the lens of the thoracoscope.

4.2.2. Contact Sapphire Tip™ Nd: YAG Laser

The Nd: YAG laser (Fig. 39) is newer than the CO$_2$ laser and more expensive. It is a powerful tool and has much deeper penetration of the tissues than the CO$_2$ laser. This laser is not absorbed by water and is color-sensitive; thus, when it hits white tissues, very little reaction occurs. Nd: YAG laser is delivered through a quartz fiber which makes the operation easier than the CO$_2$ laser. It, too, is invisible and needs to be mixed with a red He-Ne laser. A high-output Nd: YAG laser system (e.g. 100 watts) is rarely needed and a 40 watt apparatus is used in thoracoscopy. The primary use of the Nd: YAG laser is for the vaporization of malignant tissue and hemostasis, for which 25 to 35 watts of free beam Nd: YAG laser are used. A contact sapphire tip™ (Fig. 40) (SLT Surgical Laser Technology, Oaks, PA, USA) is designed to modify the delivery of Nd: YAG laser beams. There are more than a dozen different shapes of sapphire tips available. SLT's contact sapphire tip™ is found to be very useful in treating PCCs of the lungs. Type II apical bullae can be ablated very effectively with this probe. Since it is possible to feel

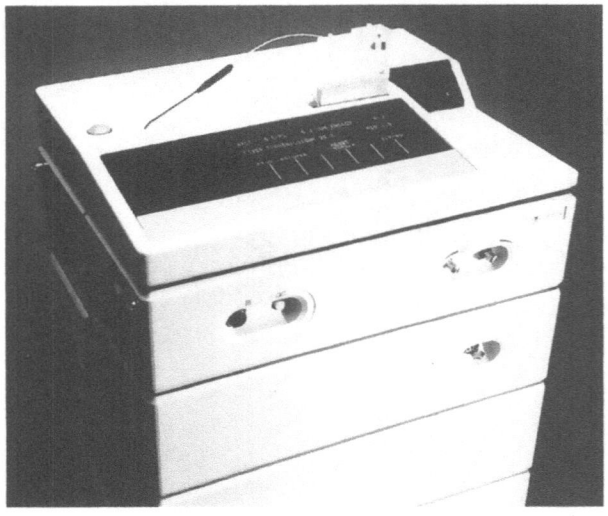

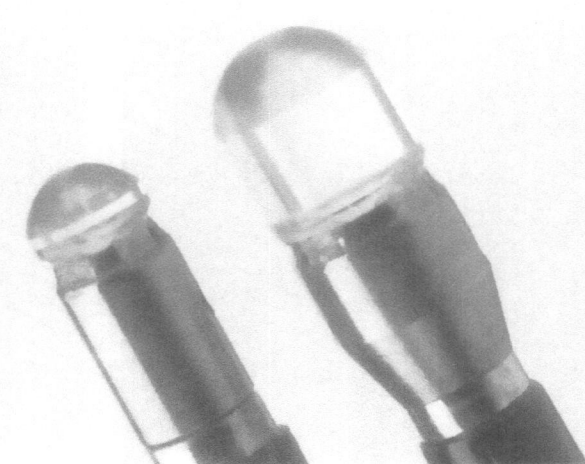

Fig. 39. Nd: YAG Unit (SLT)

Fig. 40. Contact sapphire tip (SLT)

the consistency of the tissues with this probe, one can ablate the bullae until the normal lung tissue is felt.

5. Anesthesia

General anesthesia with double-lumen endobronchial intubation (Robert-Shaw) is used in all patients. A pressure-controlled ventilator/anesthesia machine with servo mechanisms (Model 900C, Siemens, Piscataway, New Jersey, USA) is used in all cases. During thoracoscopy, we use a continuous positive airway pressure (CPAP) of 5 mmHg routinely for the ipsilateral (upper side) lung. This helps identify air leaks. Completely collapsed lungs are difficult to inspect and even slight inflation is a great help in locating the pathology. Even with CPAP, a lobe where large bronchopleural fistulae have been created by laser ablation tends to remain collapsed. Therefore, during the laser ablation of PPCs, the lung is inflated every 20 to 30 min to check for air leaks and also to relieve atelectasis. The amount of air leaks are recorded. The Siemens 900C can compensate for the loss of gas volume from leaking bullae and indicate the amount of air leaks quantitatively. Its fully computerized monitors are essential for high-risk patients with compromised pulmonary function. An Indwelling arterial line and a Swan-Ganz catheter (either oximetric or regular) are used routinely in patients

with COPD. For young patients with spontaneous pneumothorax, only a pulse oximeter is used.

The blue cuff of the endobronchial tube tends to slip out during the thoracoscopy and its position must be checked by the bronchoscope as needed. For this purpose, a video display is not necessary and the anesthesiologist simply uses a direct vision bronchoscope. When we are working on the left upper lobe and the balloon cuff of the endobronchial tube is obstructing the left upper lobe bronchus, there is no air leak. If no air leaks are found, the CPAP is removed to see if the left upper lobe completely collapses. If it does not, then the position of the blue cuff must be checked by a flexible bronchoscope. In this way, a falsenegative result for air leaks can be avoided. Cooperation between the anesthesiologist and surgeon is mandatory for satisfactory thoracoscopy.

6. Techniques

6.1. Positioning and preparation

The patient is placed in a full lateral position and the skin is prepared as for conventional thoracotomy. Drapes with deep pockets on both sides are used in order to hold the tubing, cables and instruments needed for thoracoscopic surgery.

6.2. Chest entry

A 15 mm (= circumference of a 10 mm trocar) skin incision is made in the posterior axillary line at the 5 th intercostal space. A 10 mm trocar with a blunttip obturator is inserted, while the ipsilateral lung is collapsed with a CPAP of 5 mm Hg using compressed air. The rigid thoracoscope is inserted into the trocar and the entire thoracic cavity inspected. A second 10 mm trocar hole is made at either the 4th or 5th intercostal space in the anterior axillary line, depending on the procedure within the chest cavity. Through this trocar, an operating instrument is inserted. If another instrument needs to be inserted, a 5 mm trocar is placed. Since smaller trocars can be replaced with larger trocars any time, the initial trocar should be 5 mm.

6.3. Lysis of adhesions

Fibrous adhesions are frequently encountered and must be freed to inspect the entire lung surface. An exception may be spontaneous pneumothorax in patients with severe emphysema and ruptured bullous emphysema. If a limited procedure, e.g. just to seal the leaking bullae, is elected, the trocar is inserted directly into the area and the ruptured bullae are sealed with the carbon dioxide laser. If, however, definitive treatment of the underlying diffuse bullous emphysema is contemplated, all adhesions are freed.

6.4. Techniques of ablating blebs or emphysematous bullae

In order to achieve a high success rate, we must master all the available techniques. These include; electrocautery, CO_2 laser, contact sapphire tip™ Nd: Yag laser probe, Endoloop™ (Ethicon Inc, Cincinnati, Ohio), Endo-GIA™ (United Surgical Corporation, Norwalk, Connecticut, USA), and suture ligation technique (Table 3).

6.4.1. Electrocautery

Blebs can be effectively ablated by the electrocautery without difficulty. A ruptured bleb is usually not visible as a hole, but is always covered with fibrin or accompanied by a small amount of parenchymal hemorrhage when very recent. The air leaks from ruptured blebs can be easily identified by squirting normal saline over the area while the lung is partially inflated by CPAP. The electrocautery at low energy is applied to the ruptured bleb until the air leaks stop. In order to prevent recurrence, all visible blebs must be ablated by the same technique and then the air

Table 3. Recommended techniques in treating spontaneous pneumothorax

Techniques	PPCs
Electrocautery	Blebs
Contact tip Nd: YAG laser	Type II & III
CO_2 laser	Type II & III
Endo-GIA 30	Blebs & type II
Endoloop	Small air leaks
Suture	Any air leaks not controlled by any of the above

leak is tested by inflating the ipsilateral lung to 20 mmHg. If air leaks are noticed, the electrocautery is re-applied. No leaks should be present at 20 mmHg airway pressure on completion of the thoracoscopic ablation produre. It the leak cannot be stopped, then a PDSII Endoloop™ is applied.

6.4.2. CO_2 Laser

Type II bullae cannot be effectively ablated by the electrocautery. In my personal experience, the failure rate of electrocautery for type II bullae was approximately 15 %. The CO_2 laser is more effective than the electrocautery. The CO_2 laser beams are delivered at 2 to 6 watts in a continuous wave mode to the internal surface of the bullae as well as the outside. In general, a ruptured type II bulla can be identified as a hole. If the hole is sealed with the CO_2 laser, it may recur [6] since the hole may be just the tip of an iceberg. This occurred in early experience. This complication can be prevented by opening the type II bullae down to the border with the normal lung and applying the CO_2 laser to the base.

Ruptured type III bullae in patients with COPD can be sealed off by the CO_2 laser. The low-energy laser beams are gently applied to the surrounding areas to bring the tissues inward to seal the air leaks by welding the lung tissues. If a definitive treatment rather than just sealing air leaks is contemplated, the patient is prepared as for the elective treatment of diffuse bullous emphysema.

For the treatment of diffuse bullous emphysema causing dyspnea, all type III bullae are shrunk by the CO_2 laser. Since some areas of the bullae are very thin, maximally defocused laser at 2 watts is used. Discoloration of the bullae to white to yellow indicates an adequate power density of 120 to 150 watts/cm^2. If the tissue becomes charred, the energy level is too high. If the bulla wall is perforated by the laser, the hole is closed by sutures.

6.4.3. Sapphire Contact Tip^PM Nd: YAG Laser (Fig. 40)

The sapphire contact tip™ Nd: YAG laser probe can be used for the treatment of type II bullae. A round sapphire tip is recommended for this purpose and the laser energy is set at 12-16 watts. A disadvantage of this technique is that the tip tends to stick to the bullae. The advantage is that one can feel the consistency of the bullae, so that all type II bullae can be ablated until the normal lung is felt at the junction zone. Also, the bulla walls become more rigid with the laser contraction. After the entire bullae have been ablated by the contact tip probe, the air leak is tested by squirting normal saline while the lung is inflated to 20 mmHg. If a leak is identified, the ablation procedure is repeated. If the air leak cannot be controlled with the laser alone, an Endoloop or suture is applied.

6.4.4. Endoloop™ ligation

Endoloop™ is a very useful tool in the management of spontaneous pneumothorax; nevertheless, it should be used with caution. It comes in three materials: chromic, Vicryl and PDSII. I prefer PDSII over the others. The tissue mass to be ligated should be 0.5 to 1 cm³. The ligature should not be applied to a flat surface because it may slip off when the lung is inflated, while if a large mass is ligated the tissue may undergo necrosis. These complications can be prevented by placing a figure-8 suture. A third trocar (5 mm) is inserted in the mid-clavicular line and fourth intercostal space through which a grasping probe is inserted. The Endoloop™ is inserted through the second trocar and the grasping forceps is passed through the open loop to grasp the apex of the lung. After the Endoloop™ is tightened, the air leak is again tested. If the point of leakage has been missed by the first Endoloop, another is applied. If the mass ligated by the Endoloop is larger than 1 cm³, it should be excised and a suture ligature applied. If the Endoloop is applied to a flat surface, it may slip off when the lung is fully expanded, and a suture ligature should be applied.

6.4.5. Stapling

Endo-GIA™ is another useful tool for apical type II bullae. This device is passed through a 12/13 mm disposable trocar. For apical type II bullae, the trocar is placed at the fourth intercostal space and the anterior axillary line. After the apex is freed, it is brought towards the stapler. A gauge is first applied to the tissues to make sure that the tissues to be stapled can be passed between the two blades of the gauge. If the tissues are thicker than the gauge, the Endo-GIA should not be used. If the line of stapling exceeds 3 cm, a second or third cartridge is loaded and the stapler is reapplied to complete stapling and cutting. Although this is a very useful device, it has some shortcomings. It is often difficult to apply due to the awkward angle. This problem can be solved, at least in part, by placing an Endoloop on the apex and pulling it toward the trocar hole where the Endo-GIA is inserted. Also, the tissues are frequently too thick to be stapled. If this is the case, one can start with either a CO_2 or contact Nd: YAG laser probe to cut the tissue thin and finish up with the Endo-GIA. If the Endo-GIA is applicable, it can certainly shorten the operating time considerably. It should be emphasized, however, that staplers are contraindicated for type III bullae since air leaks from staple holes are uncontrollable. Since the base of type II bullae is healthy lung tissue, air leaks from the staple holes are not a problem in young patients with type II bullae.

6.4.6. Suture ligation

If the Endoloop™ is applied to a tissue mass larger than 1 cm³, the tissue may undergo necrosis. Therefore, it should be excised and a suture placed. Also, after laser ablation of large type II apical bullae or type III bullae, if air leaks are present, they must be closed by sutures. I use a 4-0 PDSII suture with an SH needle (Ethicon Inc) or similar suture. A half-circle needle cannot be passed through a 10 mm trocar. Therefore, the needle is slightly straightened to about 3/4 of a circle. The sharp point is grasped with an endoscopic needle-holder and the needle is inserted into the 10 mm trocar. Another endoscopic needle-holder is inserted through a different 10 mm trocar to catch the needle. Bi manual coordination is critical in suturing technique. The currently available endoscopic needle-holder is unsatisfactory but it is expected that a satisfactory needle-holder will soon become available. If the endoscopic model is not available, a long regular needle-holder is used. First, the 10 mm trocar is removed and the chest-wall hole enlarged to one to two fingers breadths, depending on the distance between the target and the skin. Then the needle-holder is inserted to see if can be moved freely to suture the target. If this is satisfactory, the needle is inserted through the other trocar, and must be grasped as soon as it emerges from the trocar. Frequently, the ribs restrict the needle-holder and it may not be possible to open its jaws widely, but one should be able to open them just enough to release the needle. With this technique, it is possible to perform complicated suturing, such as continuous sutures with double rows for plication of large type III bullae. When a true endoscopic needle-holder becomes available, it will be unnecessary to enlarge the trocar hole.

References (see page 53)

Laser treatment of pseudopneumocysts of the lung

A. Wakabayashi

1. Spontaneous pneumothorax

Although spontaneous pneumothorax occurs at any age, the majority of patients are younger than 40 years of age [15-26, 29-30, 32-37]. Common initial symptoms are sudden onset of chest or back pain followed by shortness of breath. The diagnosis can be easily made by a chest X-ray film. Usually the patient receives a chest tube with continuous suction [14]. Approximately 70-80 % of the patients respond to tube thoracostomy and the pneumothorax resolves within a few days. However, a substantial number of patients develop recurrence [25, 26]. If the air leaks persist for more than 5 days, the patient usually will receive some form of invasive treatment, such as chemical sclerosing treatment (pleurodesis) [8-10, 27, 28], pleurectomy [32-36] or thoracotomy and partial lung resection [37]. Spontaneous pneumothorax in elderly patients carries a substantial morbidity and mortality rate and will be discussed separately [38, 39]. The most common underlying cause of spontaneous pneumothorax is a ruptured bleb [40]. The reason why a PPC ruptures without any obvious cause is not entirely clear. The most common cause of spontaneous pneumothorax requiring partial lung resection is type II bullae. Spontaneous pneumothorax may be caused by ruptured bronchogenic carcinoma [41] or other causes [42]. The treatment of these rare cases should be determined individually.

1. 1. Traditional treatment of spontaneous pneumothorax

1.1.1. Conservative treatment

The traditional conservative treatment is bed rest [29, 30]. If the amount of pneumothorax is less than 15 % and the patients do not have dyspnea, they can be observed as outpatients without chest tubes. If the amount of pneumothorax is greater than 15 %, it may take several days or weeks [29] for the pneumothorax to resolve by bed rest alone, which is impractical. Needle aspiration of air is ineffective. If the patients remain dyspneic or complain of chest-shoulder pain, a chest tube should be placed.

1.1.2. Tube thoracostomy

Tube thoracostomy [14, 15] is a standard treatment for spontaneous pneumothorax, and a simple but not entirely safe procedure. Frequently, it is done by a novice without proper supervision. Common complications are improper selection of the site of insertion, too large an incision for a small tube, hematoma of the chest wall, hemothorax due to laceration of the intercostal vessels, perforation of the lung or bullae, etc. In general, only a small-caliber tube is necessary for aspiration of air. A 12 F tube is adequate in most cases, and rarely more than a 20 F tube required. A convenient chest tube insertion kit is commercially available, e.g. Cook™ (Fig. 41) (Cook Inc, Bloomington, Indiana, USA) and Thora-Guide™ (Fig. 42) (Gish Medical, Santa Ana, California, USA). After placement of the chest tube, it is connected to a Pleurovac™ (Fig. 43) (Deknatel, Fall River, MA, USA) or similar device for continuous suction.

If the amount of air leak is small, the patient can be treated as an outpatient after the chest tube is connected to a flutter valve (Heimlich) [31] (Fig. 41). If the lung fails to re-expand with the Heimlich valve, however, the patient requires active suction on the tube. Continuous suction on the Pleurovac™ is maintained at 20 cm of water util the air leaks cease.

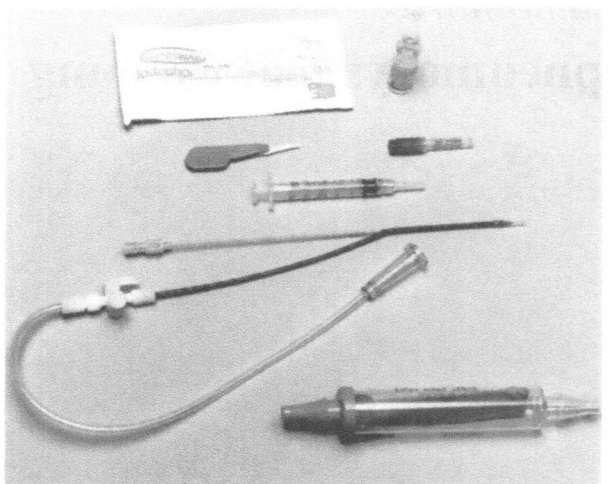

41

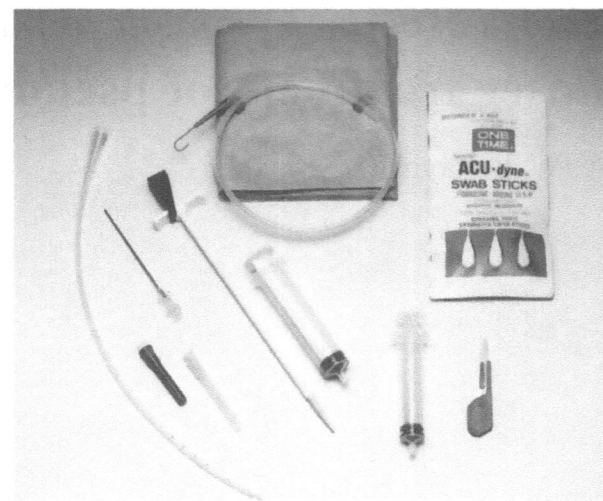

42

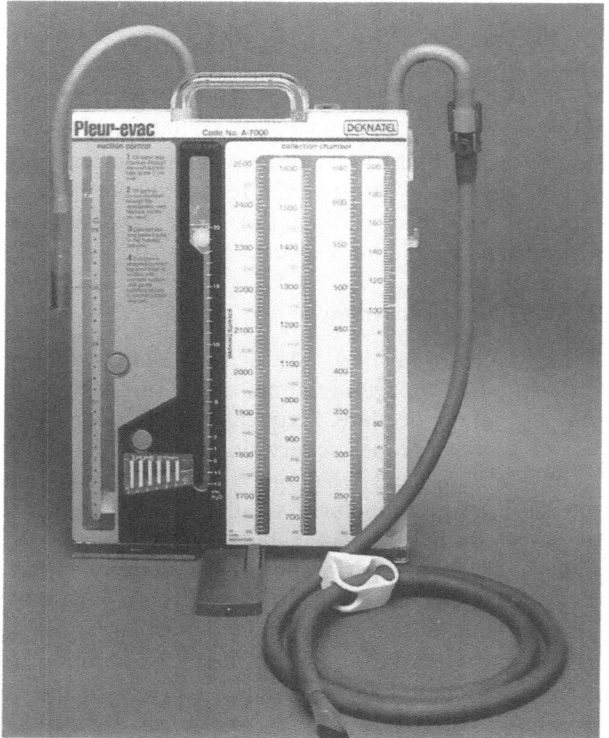

43

Fig. 41. Cook chest tube insertion kit with Heimlich valve

Fig. 42. Thora-Guide chest tube insertion kit, 12 Fr (Gish Medical)

Fig. 43. Pleurevac (Deknatel)

1.1.3. Chemical pleurodesis

Many chemical irritants have been used to induce acute inflammation of the pleura in order to sclerose the pleura. Talc powder [27, 28] and tetracycline [8] are the most common. Tetracycline was removed from the market in the United States in 1991. The instillation of any chemical irritant causes excruciating pain and its success rate is low. Thoracoscopy of patients who had previous chemical pleurodesis after they developed recurrent spontaneous pneumothorax showed that many had either no adhesions or only a few adhesions. My opinion may be biassed because, if the pleurodesis was complete, the patients would not have required thoracoscopy but this observation was made quite frequently. If the pleurodesis is effective, and the patients require thoracostomy or thoracoscopy in the future, the pleural adhesions will make it technically very difficult. For these reasons, chemical pleurodesis should be reserved for poor-risk patients who cannot tolerate general anesthesia.

1.1.4. Pleurectomy and pleural abrasion

Surgical pleurectomy [32-36] is the counterpart of chemical pleurodesis. It is carried out through a thoracotomy, usually in conjunction with partial lung resection. Some surgeons induce pleural abrasion by scraping the pleura with a gauze swab at the time of thoracotomy [15]. Surgical pleurectomy and pleural abrasion are more effective than chemical pleurodesis but carry a substantial morbidity, the most common complication being hemothorax [16]. They should therefore be regarded as indirect and adjuvant treatments. Surgical pleurectomy or pleural abrasion for recurrent spontaneous pneumothorax should be unnecessary following definitive thoracoscopic treatment provided all PPCs are thoroughly ablated.

1.1.5. Thoracotomy and lung resection

Thoracotomy and partial lung resection are the most reliable treatment for persistent or recurrent spontaneous pneumothorax in young patients [15-26, 32-37]. It carries a very low mortality and the recurrence rate is nearly zero. However, thoracotomy carries a significant morbidity. It is the most painful incision of the body wall and recovery after thoracotomy requires several weeks. In contrast to thoracotomy in young patients, thoracotomy in elderly patients with severe COPD carries a high mortality rate [38-39]. Although some authors reported excellent results in this group of patients, they still present serious problems. This will be discussed later.

1. 2. Thoracoscopic treatment of spontaneous pneumothorax

1.2.1. Background

The most reliable treatment is thoracotomy and partial resection of the PPC-containing lung and the result of any other treatments should be compared against it. The recurrence rate after partial lung resection is nearly zero, but it is a painful operation and recuperation takes several weeks. In addition, it carries a substantial risk among elderly patients with chronic obstructive pulmonary disease (COPD). Whenever I opened a chest to perform a partial lung resection, I noticed that the portion of the lungs involved was rather small and usually confined to the apex. Frequently there were small blebs in other parts of the lungs. When the electrocautery was applied to these blebs, they shrank instantly and disappeared. From this observation, I envisaged that patients with spontaneous pneumothorax could be treated without opening the chest, using a Jacobaeus thoracoscope. I found an old Jacobaeus thoracoscope [1] in the storage room and, in 1971, I tried this concept in a 17-year-old girl who had persistent spontaneous pneumothorax. Under general anesthesia, I inspected the apex of the lung. No hole was found in her lung but there were several apical blebs with yellow fibrin material adherent to them. I cauterized this area with a hot-tip cautery probe. The air leaks stopped in two days and she did very well. In the same year, I treated four additional patients with this technique and the outcome was equally successful [5]. Despite this early success, I was not certain whether it was the thoracoscopic cauterization that sealed the air leaks or whether they would have closed spontaneously. Another question was whether this procedure could prevent future recurrence. At that time, I thought this was the first successful application of thoracoscopy in the treatment of spontaneous pneumothorax but later I found a short description of this technique by Waterman in the discussion of Crenshaw's publication in 1950 [2]. The old original Jacobaeus thoracoscope was misplaced and never found again.

Thoracoscopy is simply an alternative to open thoracotomy to gain access to the intrathoracic organs through small openings. Theoretically, with appropriate instruments, nearly all the procedures traditionally performed through open thoracotomy can be performed through thoracoscopy. In addition, thoracoscopy and laser thoracoscopy have opened a new horizon in managing PPCs of the lungs. My techniques of treating PPCs, causing spontaneous pneumothorax or diffuse bullous emphysema, are essentially different from the traditional treatment. Over the past 21 years, I have found that PPCs of the lungs do not require excision but can simply be ablated by electrocautery [5] or laser [6].

1.2.2. Techniques

The successful thoracoscopic management of spontaneous pneumothorax requires mastery of all available thoracoscopic techniques (Table 1). In general, blebs are ablated by electrocautery and type II apical bullae by either CO_2 laser or contact sapphire tip™ Nd: Yag laser. If any air leaks are noticed after laser ablation, either Endoloop™, Endo-GIA™, or sutures will be added. No leaks should be present upon completion of the procedure at an airway pressure of 20 mmHg. Pleurectomy or pleural abrasion should not be added, since these are ineffective, unnecessary and painful. In treating young and otherwise healthy patients, I prefer not to leave any metallic materials such as staples or surgical clips inside the chest which are demonstrable on chest X-ray films. This is, however, a matter of personal preference. A small chest tube (12 or 16 F) is inserted through one of the trocar holes and connected to a Pleurovac™ (Fig. 43) to evacuate residual air. The Valsalva maneuver cannot evacuate the residual air completely and should not be used. Once the lung is fully re-expanded and no air leaks are noted, the chest tube is removed. I prefer latex rubber tubing to Silastic tubing because it is easier to milk the tubing to check a minute amount of air leaks. Most young patients can be discharged within 24 hours after surgery.

1.2.3. Results (Table 2)

In addition to 5 patients treated in 1971, 116 patients were treated by thoracoscopy from 1987 to 1991. 38 patients had ruptured blebs, 59 ruptured type II bullae, 16 ruptured type III bullae and 3 had other causes. Electrocautery was successful in 95 % and unsuccessful in 5 %. The causes of failure (Table 3) were inappropriate thoracoscope optic/video systems in 6, inability of electrocautery to seal air leaks in 1, technical error in sealing air leaks in 1, a slipped metal clip in 1 and slowghing after ligation of excessive tissue in 1. In early series, the video camera often had to be removed from the thoracoscope to view directly through the thoracoscope. I also used a split-beam video camera with a prism, so as to see through the thoracoscope while the procedure was recorded on a video recorder. As the optic/video systems improved, direct vision thoracoscopy became rarely necessary.

For ruptured type II bullae, electrocautery had a high failure rate due to inability to ablate deep-seated

Table 1. Recommended techniques in treating spontaneous pneumothorax

Techniques	PPCs
Electrocautery	Blebs
Contact tip Nd: YAG laser	Type II & III
CO_2 laser	Type II & III
Endo-GIA 30	Blebs & type II
Endoloop	Small air leaks
Suture	Any air leaks not controlled by any of the above

Table 2. Clinical results

Cause	Number	Success	Failure	%
Blebs	38	36	2	5
Type II	59	55	4	7
Type III	16	13	3	19
Other*	3	2	1	33
Total	116	106	10	9

* Eosinophilic granuloma 1, Endometriosis 1, Squamous cell carcinoma 1

Table 3. Causes of failure*

Inadequate optic al systems	6
Inability to seal air laks	2
Metal clip slippage	1
Tissue necrosis by Endoloop	1

* Two of 116 patients required subsequent thoracotomy, one by an other surgeon and another by the author. All other failures were corrected by repeated thoracoscopy.

lesions. Therefore more effective sealing tools were investigated. The CO_2 laser was very effective in sealing a hole in the bulla. However, it gives a false sense of success; though no air leaks are noted on completion of the procedure the leaks restart within an hour in the recovery room. Moveover, the CO_2 laser sealed only the rupture site, leaving the underlying deep intraparenchymal bullae of type II. This problem was solved, at least in part, by opening the bullae to the base and aiming the laser beams into the internal surface of the bullae. The contact tip Nd: YAG laser probe had a higher success rate than the CO_2 laser in treating spontaneous pneumothorax. This may be because the contact tip technique was initiated only recently after the author had gained experience and the other instrumentation had improved, or because it was possible to feel the consistency of the bullae with the probe and to ablate them until the border with the normal lung was reached. A sapphire contact tip Nd: YAG laser probe was used in 27 cases. Twenty-one patients did not require any additional treatment. In 6 patients (22%), additional measures using either Endoloop, suture closure or both was required to stop the air leak completely. Of 47 patients who were treated by the CO_2 laser, 18 patients (38%) required additional Endoloop, suture closure or both. Sixteen patients developed spontaneous pneumothorax secondary to ruptured type III bullae. Thirteen were successfully treated by thoracoscopic ablation or sealing of ruptured bullae. Three required repeated thoracoscopic treatment when the first attempt failed to control air leaks. One patient with ruptured eosinophilic granulomas required repeated thoracoscopy but the CO_2 laser failed to seal the leaks. He was subsequently treated by thoracotomy and partial lung resection. A patient with catamenial spontaneous pneumothorax was treated successfully with free-beam Nd: YAG laser resection of three nodules from the right lower lobe. She did not require any stitches. One patient with a ruptured small endobronchial carcinoma of the right lower lobe and severe COPD was treated by simple suture closure since his pulmonary function was so poor that he would not tolerate lung resection.

Follow-up of these patients was relatively short, except for the first 5 patients who were treated more than 20 years ago. So far, no recurrence was noted. The success rate of thoracoscopic treatment depends on the instrumentation and experience of the surgeon. The high success rate of the past two years is due to improved optic/video systems, instruments and anesthesia, and complete ablation of all PPCs using all available methods, including staplers and suturing techniques. No air leaks should be demonstrated with the lungs inflated by manual ventilation up to 20 mm Hg upon completion of thoracoscopic surgery. From these clinical observations, it is concluded that thoracoscopic treatment of spontaneous pneumothorax is a definitive treatment of PPCs of the lung with an extremely low recurrence rate and is the treatment of choice. The next question is whether we should treat a first episode of spontaneous pneumothorax by thoracoscopy. The author has treated several first-time comers by the thoracoscopic technique. However, a prospective randomized study is required to see if this approach is medically and economically justifiable.

1.3. Treatment of ruptured diffuse bullous emphysema

Spontaneous pneumothorax due to ruptured type III bullae in patients with COPD should be mentioned separately. Simple chest tube placement alone carries

a substantial mortality rate [38, 39].The amount of air leak is quite large and may interfere with respiration, which is already severely compromised. Frequently the hypoxemia cannot be corrected with a high-flow supplementary oxygen. Sixteen thoracoscopic operations were performed on 15 such patients. The first 6 patients were treated by minimal laser surgery, i.e. only the ruptured bullae were sealed with the CO_2 laser without freeing the adhesions, if any. Repeated procedure was required in 3 patients. One of these developed recurrent spontaneous pneumothorax two years later and underwent a second thoracoscopic treatment. This patient and 10 subsequent patients were given definitive treatment; all adhesions were freed and all bullae ablated with the laser. None required repeated procedures and all did well. In contrast to type II bullae, staplers are contraindicated for type III bullae since air leaks from staple holes are numerous and tend to persist for a very long time. Computed tomography of the lungs is helpful in planning treatment for this group of patients prior to surgery.

2. Diffuse bullous emphysema

2.1. Traditional treatment of diffuse bullous emphysema

Diffuse bullous emphysema is commonly seen among elderly chronic smokers or ex-smokers and in patients with other acquired or congenital disorders [43-45]. The inspired air enters the bullae but may be trapped therein, causing an increased pressure inside the bullae that is higher than the intraalveolar pressure. These tense bullae behave like a localised tension pneumothorax and interfere with the function of the adjacent lung tissue. On a dynamic Imatron scan, it has been observed that a large tense bulla of the right upper lobe moves like a pendulum during inspiration and expiration without changing its size and impinges upon the right main bronchus, thus obstructing the airway. As a compensatory mechanism, the body will respond by expanding the volume of the chest cavity by changing the vertical position of the ribs to a horizontal position, increasing the anterior-posterior diameter of the chest, and depressing and flattening the diaphragm. This process takes many years during which time the patients with COPD remain relatively symptom-free. As the bullae continue to increase in size, the body will no longer be able to increase the volume of the chest cavity. From this point, the dyspnea on exertion starts to worsen rapidly [45]. The bullae may rupture, causing spontaneous pnemothorax [38], or they may become infected but the most common sequel is acute respiratory failure due to bronchitis or lobar pneumonia. There is no definitive treatment for diffuse bullous emphysema, only symptomatic relief by bronchodilators. Occasionally, surgical removal of bullae [46-58] or intracavitary insufflation with sclerosing agents [59-62] may result in dramatic improvement of lung function. However, experience indicates that patients with severe emphysema [63-65] or alpha-1 antitrypsin deficiency [66] respond poorly to surgical treatment. Only patients with isolated compressive bullae and crowding of the adjacent vasculature [67-69] have shown significant improvement of lung function. Consequently, surgical bullectomy is of benefit to only very few patients and is not applicable to the majority.

2.2. Laser thoracoscopic treatment of diffuse bullous emphysema

2.2.1. Background

When treating patients with spontaneous pneumothorax with the carbon dioxide (CO_2) laser in 1989, I found large bullae (retrospectively, type I) not related to spontaneous pneumothorax in two. Out of curiosity, I fired the laser beam at them and to my surprise they shrank almost instantly. Based on this observation, I developed a thoracoscopic method to ablate pulmonary bullae using a low-energy CO_2 laser that does not require open thoracotomy. The preliminary result was published in 1991 [11].

2.2.2. Patient selection

Patient selection is based on 1) dyspnea at rest or with minimal exertion, and 2) chest radiographs or computed tomographic (CT) lung scans demonstrating bullous lung disease. In some patients, tightness and chest pain on minimal exertion, mimiking angina pectoris, were the main symptoms. In addition to a routine physical examination and laboratory testing, complete pulmonary function tests including plethysmography [67-70] and treadmill tests, using a modified protocol designed for emphysema patients [71-72], were obtained before the laser treatment. In the early phase of the study, three extremely sick patients were transferred from other hospitals. We were unable to perform these tests for these moribund patients. One patient died two weeks after surgery and the others two within four months after discharge from the hospital. We therefore no longer accept patients directly from the intensive care units of other hospitals for surgery.

Instead, we place them on a pulmonary rehabilitation program to optimize their condition prior to surgery. With this new protocol, one patient had successful bilateral procedures and another died during preoperative rehabilitation. Careful cardiac evaluation is essential. Emphysema patients do not exert themselves due to shortness of breath, and frequently any underlying ischemic heart disease is not recognized. Some patients develop electrocardiographic changes suggestive of ischemia or dysrhythmia. These are subjected to dobutamine echocardiography and if the result suggests myocardial ischemia coronary angiography should be performed. One of the patients so selected was found to have more than 90 % right coronary artery stenosis and underwent percutaneous transluminal coronary artery angioplasty (PTCA), which was complicated by hypotension requiring partial cardiopulmonary bypass via percutaneously placed cannulae. He underwent laser thoracoscopy subsequently without incident. Two patients developed severe hypotension immediately after the induction of anesthesia and the surgery was canceled. One of them had previous coronary artery bypass surgery.

Surgery was canceled and they were studies by coronary angiography. One of them had normal coronary arteries and the other had patent grafts. Subsequently both of them underwent the laser bullectomy without problems. Currently we are evaluating another screening processes. During the routine preoperative assessment of the bullous disease of the lung by means of fast scanner computed tomography (Imatron™), the calcium deposits on the coronary arteries were checked by the radiologist. If significant deposits were demonstrated on the left main coronary artery or proximal three vessels, the patients were subjected to coronary angiography. Only one of six patients with positive calcium deposits was found to have significant coronary artery occlusive disease. This patient underwent PTCA, which was complicated by dissection of the left anterior descending coronary artery and required repeated PTCA. Subsequently she underwent laser bullectomy without a problem. It appears that the Imatrom™ test is too sensitive and produces too many false positive results and its clinical value is questionable. We shall continue to evaluate this technique until a final answer is reached. It is anticipated that we will encounter a patient who has severe diffuse bullous emphysema with significant occlusive coronary artery disease. Each case should be evaluated and handled on individual basis.

In general, the conventional CT films are adequate for screening. If it is difficult to identify the bullae amenable to laser shrinkage, we use the Imatron. Not only is this more sensitive than conventional CT, but

Imatron with dynamic scanning also demonstrates the dynamic action of the bullae which has never been possible before. The size of the bullae remains unchanged during inspiration and expiration, indicating that the intraluminal tension does not change during expiration. Some bullae showed pendulum motion and clearly compressed the main bronchus during expiration. More detailed analysis of the data obtained from these studies will shed light on the mechanism of respiratory impairment in emphysema patients.

Many patients are on continuous oxygen. Neither hypoxemia nor hypercapnia is in itself a contraindication to laser bullectomy. Many patients had a clinical diagnosis of cor pulmonale. Currently there is no reliable noninvasive technique to measure the right ventricular pressure. Some patients had a history of spontaneous pneumothorax and tube thoracostomy. This does not preclude laser bullectomy. Patients who have had previous thoracotomy and lobectomy for any reason should be excluded.

2.2.3. Techniques

Early cases were treated with an NIIR surgical system (NIIC USA, Inc, Redwood City, CA). The majority of patients were treated with a Coherent unit (Coherent, Palo Alto, CA). Since the CO_2 laser travels through articulated arms, its alignment becomes frequently incorrect and power is lost. The power setting used varied from 2 to 33 watts, but when the alignment is correct, 2 to 4 watts are adequate. In order to direct the CO_2 laser beams as perpendicularly as possible to the bullae, the articulated arms must often be pulled down almost to a horizontal position. This may disalign the laser beam which can be prevented by a fixed-focus waveguide. A laser scope with a Gallerian focusing device (Olympus) is capable of adjusting the focusing of the laser beams. Using this device, the laser beam is maximally defocused. This increases the speed of the procedure and may also reduce the possibility of perforation. Another advantage of the laser scope is that the CO_2 laser beam with a helium-neon aiming beam is in the visual field and the laser can be fired immediately on seeing the bullae. The disadvantage of the laser scope is that the connection tends to become loose and the alignment becomes off, a frequent problem when the laser scope is held horizontally. The disadvantage of the waveguide is that its focus is fixed and the probe has to be retracted when the spot size needs to be enlarged.

However, it can remain in correct alignment in a horizontal position. The CO_2 laser is safe and easy to use, especially at a low energy level, since the penetration is extremely shallow.

The CO_2 laser is fired at the bullae while it is monitored on the video screen. The power density of the laser has many variables and the only reliable way to monitor it is to watch the color changes in the tissues. The optimal power density produces white to yellow discoloration. If the bulla walls become black, the energy level should be lowered, otherwise the laser will perforate the bullae. If the laser hits the bullous wall tangentially, the power density becomes less. Therefore, the lateral surfaces of the bullae should be ablated by the waveguide which is passed through perpendicularily to the laserscope. Large bullae on the surface of the major fissures are common and need to be shrunk by this lateral approach. Since the lower pulmonary lobe artery lies in the major fissure, extreme caution must be exercised in this area. For type I bullae, it is excised. As soon as a hole is made in the dome of the bulla, the bulla collapses and can be pulled out of the trocar hole. The bulla wall is then excised outside the chest while its base is watched by the thoracoscope placed inside the chest. A few communicating holes with the bronchial systems are identified and closed with the laser, followed by suture closure. Type III bullae are simply shounk/ If perforations are made, the inner surfaces of the bullae are thermocoagulated by the laser. If air leaks can not be controlled, sutures are applied preferably an absorbable 4-0 PDSII suture with a long and thin needle (SH). Occasionally, pledgets are necessary. Autogenous tissues, e.g. pleura, are preferred to synthetic materials for this purpose.

2.2.4. Post-operative care

The patients are maintained on a mechanical ventilator until adequate oxygenation can be achieved through a nasal oxygen cannula. Increased sputum production may delay weaning. In general, pulmonary function is worse for the first two days than the immediate preoperative status. It reaches the preoperative level in 7 to 10 days and continues to improve for the first three to five months. The chest tubes are left in place until air leaks stop. Physical therapy and pulmonary rehabilitation are instituted at an early postoperative stage. If ventilatory support is required for more than 48 hours, a nasogastric tube feeding is commenced on day two to maintain positive calorie intake. Cephalosporin is used intravenously for two to three days. After the patient is weaned off the ventilator, he/she is transferred out of the intensive care unit, where he/she undergoes progressive rehabilitation.

2.2.5. Results (Table 4)

Fifty seven laser thoracoscopies were carried out in the treatment of diffuse bullous emphysema causing dyspnea in 44 patients (37 males and 7 females) over a period from May 1989 to December 1991. Mean age was 61 years old. Only three patients had type I bullae and the majority of them had type III bullae. During this period, 5 patients underwent bilateral laser thoracoscopies ; 3 elective and 2 urgent. Many complications were encountered. The most common complication was persistent air leaks and repeated thoracoscopies were required to control persistent air leaks from bronchopleural fistulae in 4 patients. Sub-cutaneous emphysema was also a common complication which was relieved by a second anterior chest tube. One patient required thoracotomy for hemorrhage. This patient had extensive adhesions and the bleeding was diffuse from the chest wall. Three patients died, the operative mortality rate being 5 % (Table 5). The causes of deaths were acute myocardial infarction in a patient who had previous coronary artery bypass grafting, pneumonia and sepsis in an elderly woman who was on a high dose of prednisone for many years before surgery, and liver failure in an alcoholic patient with liver cirrhosis. One patient died within 2 weeks after discharge 7 days after surgery. She apparently developed pneumonia of the opposite lung and refused to see a doctor. When finally readmitted, she was in septic shock and died in a few days. Pneumonia of the opposite lung is a serious complication and not uncommon. The first patient in our series, a 75-years-old male, had this complication three weeks after surgery but was – successfully – managed by vigorous antibiotic treatment. He underwent laser bullectomy of the opposite side three months later and enjoyed almost normal life for two years but died two years later of stroke. Three late deaths were also due to pneumonia of the opposite side, which occurred within two to four months of discharge. Two of these three patients were moribund and transferred from the intensive care units of other hospitals ; although they survived surgery, they required prolonged hospitalisation. After discharge, they developed pneumonia of the opposite lungs and died. The third patient was not considered a high-risk patient. After surgery, the bullae of the opposite side became extremely enlarged and crossed the midline. He could not be weaned from the ventilator for a long time and required tracheostomy. He died at home two months later due to pneumonia of the opposite lung. Retrospectively, this patient should have had the opposite side operated when he could not be weaned off the ventilator. In another patient, such an aggressive approach was very successful.

Early in the series, we noticed a very peculiar complication. Within 24 to 48 hours after laser bullectomy, the patient developed hypoxemia and the

Table 4. Diffuse bullous emphysema : clinical data

Number of Patients :	44
Sex : Male	37
Female	7
Age (mean) :	61
Type : I	3
III	42
Number of operations :	57
Number of bilateral operations	5
Repeated thoracoscopies (BPF)	4
Thoracotomy (hemorrhage)	1

Table 5. Causes of death

A. Hospital Deaths (3)	
Respiratory failure	1
Acute myocardial infarction	1
Liver failure	1
B. early deaths (1)	
Pneumonia	1
C. late deaths (4)	
Respiratory failure	3
Stroke	1

chest film showed diffuse infiltrates of the lungs. The first patient required reintubation two days after surgery. This phenomenon was also noted in a patient who had prolonged spontaneous pneumothorax and was treated by CO_2 laser. The laser time was short and only the ruptured superior segment bullae were sealed with the CO_2 laser. Her chest film showed a typical white lung pattern, although she had no clinical evidence of hypoxemia. This radiologic finding is not necessarily associated with hypoxemia, as in this patient. Initially, we thought this might be due to rapid expansion of the lungs because it appeared to be similar to re-expansion edema. Therefore, in a couple of patients, we did staged operations, several days appart. This had no effect and was quickly abandoned. We then adopted a policy that vacuum suction was not applied for the first several hours and the chest tube was connected only to an underwater seal. However, this did not change the picture. As we gained more experience, this picture was seen less often. The cause of this is still under investigation. One of my colleagues has been studying this phenomenon using a rabbit model and found that humoral mediators may be involved. This « white lung syndrome » is fortunately subclinical in the majority of cases. Six patients underwent bilateral procedures three and four months appart. In early experience, two patients were subjected to a two-stage operation, four to five days appart, in an attempt to prevent re-expansion interstitial pulmonary edema. This proved unsuccessful and therefore we abandoned the two-stage operation. This complication occurs in almost all patients to some degree, but fortunately is usually functionally mild and only demonstrable on chest radiographs. We have some experimental data suggesting that this complication may be humorally mediated and characteristic of the CO_2 laser. This study is still under way.

If the patients are moribund and dependent on a high dose of steroids, the risk of surgery is very high. Even they survive the operation and go home, the short-term result is poor. Therefore, these patients should not be selected for surgery. One patient was referred from other hospital but we deferred surgery. During preoperative pulmonary rehabilitation in order to optimize the patient's condition, she died of pulmonary failure. During this study periods, other six patients died while they were waiting for surgery, indicating the severity of their illness. During the past four months, 22 patients underwent laser bullectomy without deaths.

The most common complication is persistent air leaks. Perforation of bullae by the laser should be identified and sealed with the laser or suture closed during operation. This problem is often encountered in patients who are taking steroids for a long time before surgery. We try to taper down the Prednisone to an arbitrary number of 5 mg a day before surgery. However, there is no data supporting this policy.

Forty four patients are eligible for 3-month or longer follow up studies. The results indicate that all but one showed significant increase in FVC, FEV, MVV ($p < 0.001$) and treadmill tests ($p < 0.005$). There was no significant change in DLCO. The details of the data will be published in a near future. The only patient who had recurrence was found to smoke three packs of cigarettes a day. This is the youngest patient of our series and is schizophrenic. Resumption of smoking was reportedly associated with a high incidence of recurrence [69] following surgical bullectomy. Therefore, we do not accept any patients who can not refrain from smoking for two months. It has been reported that patients with anti-trypsin deficiency showed rapid recurrence and deterioration following surgical bullectomy [55, 68, 69]. This was not observed in our five patients, four of when are receiving alpha-1 antitrypsin replacement. In conclusion, thoracoscopic CO_2 laser ablation of emphysematous bullae can be carried out with a reasonable risk and offers a sustained improvement in pulmonary function and physical capacity.

References

1. Jacobaeus HC (1915) Endopleurale Operationen unter der Leitung des Thorakoskops. Beitr Z Klin Tuber 35 : 1-35
2. Crenshaw GL (1950) Etiology, treatment and surgical indications of nontuberculous, nontraumatic spontaneous pneumothorax. Dis Chest 17 : 369-387
3. Ratliff JL, Johnson N, Clever JA (1977) Pleuroscopy and cautery control of intrathoracic hemorrhage with a flexible fiberoptic bronchoscope. Chest 71 : 216-217
4. Takeno Y (1978) Un nouveau traitement du pneumothorax spontané par nébulisation d'une colle liquide sous contrôle thoracoscopique. Broncho-Pneumologie 28 : 19-28
5. Wakabayashi A (1989) Thoracoscopic ablation of blebs in the treatment of recurrent or persistent spontaneous pneumothorax. Ann Thorac Surg 48 : 651-653
6. Wakabayashi A, Brenner M, Wilson AF, Tadir Y, Berns M (1990) Thoracoscopic treatment of spontaneous pneumothorax using carbon dioxide laser. Ann Thorac Surg 50 : 786-790
7. Abyholm F, Stren G, Geiran O (1975) Spontaneous pneumothorax. Scan J Thorac Cardiovasc Surg 9 : 281-286
8. Krasnik M, Christensen B, Lalkier E, Hoeir-Madsen K, Jelnes R, Wied U (1987) Pleurodesis in spontaneous pneumothorax by means of tetracycline: Follow-up evaluation of a method. Scand J Thor Cardiovasc Surg 21 : 181-182
9. Brock RC (1948) Recurrent and chronic spontaneous pneumothorax. Thorax 3 : 88
10. Torre M, Belloni P (1989) Nd: YAG laser pleurodesis through thoracoscopy: new curative therapy in spontaneous pneumothorax. Ann Thorac Surg 47 : 887-889
11. Wakabayashi A, Brenner M, Kayaleh R, et al (1991) Thoracoscopic carbon dioxide laser treatment of bullous emphysema. Lancet 337 : 881-883
12. Terminology, definitions, and classification of chronic pulmonary emphysema and related conditions. A report of the conclusions of a CIBA guest symposium. Thorax (1959) 14 : 286-299
13. Laurenzi GA, Turing GM and Fishman AP (1962) Bullous disease of the lung. AM J Med 32 : 361-378
14. Klassen KP, Meckstroth CV (1962) Treatment of spontaneous pneumothorax: Prompt expansion with controlled thoracotomy tube suction. JAMA 182 : 1-5
15. Clark TA, Hutchinson DE, Deaner RM, Fitchett VH (1972) Spontaneous pneumothorax. Am J Surg 124 : 728-731
16. Mills M, Baisch BF (1965) Spontaneous pneumothorax: A series of 400 cases. Ann Thorac Surg 1 : 286-297
17. Driscoll PJ, Aronstam EM (1961) Experiences in the management of recurrent spontaneous pneumothorax. J Thorac Cardiovasc Surg 42 : 174-178
18. Lichter J, Gwyne JF (1971) Spontaneous pneumothorax in young subjects. Thorax 26 : 409-417
19. Lichter I (1974) Long-term follow-up of planned treatment of spontaneous pneumothorax. Thorax 29 : 32-37

20. Hagen RH, Reed W, Solheim K (1987) Spontaneous pneumothorax. Scand J Thorac Cardiovasc Surg 21 : 183-185

21. Lindkog GE, Halasz DA (1957) Spontaneous pneumothorax. Arch Surg 75 : 693-698

22. Mark JB, Lindkog GE (1961) Spontaneous pneumothorax with special emphasis on treatment. Conn Med 25 : 479-483

23. Shefts LM, Gilpatrick C, Swindell H et al (1954) Management of spontaneous pneumothorax. Dis Chest 26 : 273-285

24. Saha SP, Arrants JE, Kosa A, Lee WH Jr. (1975) Management of spontaneous pneumothorax. Ann Thorac Surg 19 : 561-564

25. Gobbell WG Jr, Rhea WG Jr, Nelson IA, Daniel RA Jr (1963) Spontaneous pneumothorax. J Thorac Cardiovasc Surg 46 : 331-345

26. Serementis MG (1970) The management of spontaneous pneumothorax. Chest 57 : 65-68

27. Adler RH (1968) A talc powder aerosol method for the prevention of recurrent spontaneous pneumothorax. Ann Thorac Surg 5 : 474-477

28. Nandi P (1980) Recurrent spontaneous pneumothorax. Chest 77 : 493-495

29. Hyde L (1962) Benign spontaneous pneumothorax. Ann Intern Med 56 : 746-751

30. Levy IJ (1966) Spontaneous pneumothorax: Treat-ment based on analysis of 170 episodes in 135 pa-tients. Dis Chest 49 : 529-537

31. Page A, Cossette R, Dontigny L, Levy R, Mercia C, Pelletier LC, Verdant A (1975) Spontaneous pneumothorax, outpatient management with intercostal tube drainage. Can Med Assn J 112 : 707-713

32. Gaensler EA (1956) Partial pleurectomy for recurrent spontaneous pneumothorax. Surg Gynecol Obstet 102 : 293-308

33. Thomas PA, Gebauer PW (1958) Pleurectomy for recurrent spontaneous pneumothorax J Thorac Surg 35 : 111-117

34. Thomas PA, Gebauer PW (1960) Results and complication of pleurectomy for bullous emphysema and recurrent pneumothorax. J Thorac Cardiovasc Surg 39 : 194-201

35. Askew AR (1976) Parietal pleurectomy for recurrent pneumothorax. Br J Surg 63 : 203-205

36. DesLauriers J, Beaulieu M, Despres JP, Lemieux M, Leblanc J, Desmeules M. Transaxillary pleurectomy for treatment of spontaneous pneumothorax. Ann Thorac Surg 30 : 569-574

37. Brooks JW (1973) Open thoracotomy in the management of spontaneous pneumothorax. Ann Surg 177 : 798-805

38. Shield T, Oilschlager GA (1966) Spontaneous pneumothorax in patients 40 years of age and older. Ann Thorac Surg 2 : 377-383

39. Smith WG (1964) The significance of spontaneous pneumothorax in middle life. Geriatrics 19 : 795-802

40. Withers JN, Fishback ME, Kiehl PV, Hannon JL (1964) Spontaneous pneumothorax: Suggested etiology and comparison of treatment methods. Am J Surg 108 : 772-776

41. Battaglin JW, Shallal JA, Wilcox BR (1980) Bronchogenic carcinoma presenting as spontaneous pneumothorax. Report of two cases and review of the literature. NC Med J 41 : 805

42. Crutcher RR, Waltuch Tl, Blue ME (1967) Recurring spontaneous pneumothorax associated with menstruation. J TCVS 54 : 599

43. Smith J, Alerts C and Balk AG (1978) Pneumothorax in the Ehlers-Danlos syndrome: Consequence or coincidence? Scand J Respir Dis 59 : 239-242

44. Ayers JG, Pope FM, Feidy JF et al Abnormalities of the lungs and thoracic cage in the Ehlers-Danlos syndrome. Thorax 40 : 300-305

45. Ogilvie C and Caterall M (1959) Patterns of disturbed lung function in patients with emphysematous bullae. Thorax 14 : 216-224

46. Potgieter PD, Benatar SR, Hewitson RP et al (1981) Surgical treatment of bullous lung disease. Thorax 36 : 885-890

47. Brantigan OE, Mueler E and Kress MD (1959) A surgical approach to bullous emphysema. Am Rev Resp Dis 80 : 194-204

48. Woo-Ming M, Capel LH, Belcher JR (1963) The results of treatment of large air cysts of the lung. Br J Dis Chest 57 : 79-85

49. Fain WR, Conn JH, Campbell GD et al (1967) Excision of giant pulmonary emphysematous cysts: Report of 20 cases without deaths. Surgery 62 : 552-559

50. Rogers RM, DuBois AB and Blakemore WS (1968) Effect of removal of bullae on airway conductance and conductance volume rations. J Clin Invest 47 : 2569-2579

51. Lopez-Mjano V, Kieffer RJ Jr, Marine DN, Garcia DA, Wagner HN Jr (1969) Pulmonary resection in bullous disease. Am Rev Respir Dis 99 : 554-564

52. Wesley JR, Maclead WM and Mullard KS (1972) Evaluation and surgery of bullous emphysema. J Thorac Cardiovasc Surg 63 : 945-955

53. Braun Sr, DePico GA, Birnbaum ML et al (1973) Bullae and severe generalized disease. Successful treatment with bullectomy. J Thorac Cardiovasc Surg 65 : 26-29

54. Gunstensen J, and McCormack RJ (1973) The surgical management of bullous emphysema. J Thorac Cardiovasc Surg 65 : 920-925

55. Pearson MG and Ogilvie C (1983) Surgical treatment of emphysematous bullae: Late outcome. Thorax 38 : 134-137

56. O'Brien CJ, Hughes CF, Gianoutsos P (1986) Surgical treatment of bullous emphysema. Aust NZJ Surg 56 : 241-245

57. Laros CD, Gelissen HJ, Bergstein PG et al (1986) Bullectomy for giant bullous emphysema. J Thorac Cardiovac Surg 91 : 63-70

58. Connolly JE and Wilson A (1989) The current status of surgery for bullous emphysema. J Thorac Cardiovasc Surg 97 : 351-361

59. Head JR and Avery AA. Intracavitary suction (Monaldi) in the treatment of emphysematous bullae and blebs. J Thorac Cardiovasc Surg 40 : 443-460

60. Head JM, Head IR, Hudson TR, Head JR. The surgical treatment of emphysematous blebs and localized vesicular and bullous emphysema. J Thorac Cardiovasc Surg 40 : 443-460

61. Mac Arthur AM and Fountain SW (1977) Intracavitary suction and drainage in the treatment of emphysematous bullae. Thorax 32 : 668-672

62. Venn GE, Williams PR and Goldstraw P (1988) Intracavitary drainage for bullous emphysematous lung disease: Experience with the Brompton technique. Thorax 43 : 998-1002

63. Baldwin E, Harden AA, Greene DG et al (1950) Pulmonary insufficiency. IV. A study of 16 cases of large air cysts or bullae. Medicine 29 : 169-194

64. Sieben AA, Grant AR, Kent DC et al (1957) Pulmonary cystic disease: Physiologic studies and results of resection. J Thorac Surg 33 : 185

65. Nakahara K, Kanaoka K, Ohon K et al (1983) Functional indications for bullectomy of giant bulla. Ann Thorac Surg 35 (5) : 480-487

66. Talamo RC JDA, Kahan MG et al (1968) Hereditary alpha 1-antitrypsin deficiency. N Engl J Med 278 : 345-351

67. Gaensler EA, Jederlinic PJ and Fitzgerald MX (1986) Patient work-up for bullectomy. J Thorac Imaging 1 : 75-93

68. Hughes JA, MacArthur AM, Huchison DCS, Hugh-Jones P (1984) Long-term changes in lung function after surgical treatment of bullous emphysema in smokers and exsmokers. Thorax 39 : 140-142

69. FitzGerald MX, Keelan PJ, Cugell DW et al (1974) Long-term results of surgery for bullous emphysema. J Thorac & Cardiovasc Surg 68 (4) : 556-587

70. Boushy SF, Kohen R, Billig DM, Hwiman MJ (1968) Bullous emphysema: Clinical, roentgenologic and physiologic study of 49 patients. Dis Chest 54 : 327-334

71. Tenholder MF, Jones PA, Matthews JL et al (1980) Bullous emphysema. Progressive incremental exercice testing to evaluate candidates for bullectomy. Chest 77 (6) : 802-805

72. Wasserman K and Whipp BJ (1975) Exercice physiology in health and disease. Am Rev Respir Dis 112 : 219-249

Thoracoscopic treatment of pneumothorax

Laser pleurodesis

M. Torre and P.A. Belloni

1. Introduction

The optimal treatment in spontaneous pneumothorax should achieve two different objectives:

1) radical treatment of the lung lesion that produced the air leak from the lung into the pleural space;

2) induction of a permanent pleurodesis in order to guarantee effective adhesion between the visceral and parietal pleura in order to prevent recurrences. These goals should be obtained with the least discomfort for the patient.

By 1906, different authors had proposed several methods useful in producing pleurodesis in order to avoid the potential hazards of surgery [3, 6]. Their general principle is the induction of adhesions between the visceral and parietal pleura. In such cases pleurodesis may be induced physically (by mechanical or traumatic procedures) or chemically by application of different substances able to induce an inflammatory reaction of the mesothelium that produces adhesions and fibrosis formation of a different nature. These methods can be performed through thoracostomy tubes or through thoracoscopy [5, 6].

In 1906 Spengler first attempted pleurodesis with hypertonic glucose and later with 5% silver nitrate [3]. Bethune in 1935, Singer in 1941, and Daniel in 1990 [4, 6, 7] emphasized the use of iodized talc as an effective method. Talc is a vigorous fibrogenic agent and induces an intense reaction but has been condemned because it can be extremely painful, may lead to fibrothorax, an induce talc granulomata and is sometimes associated with pleural carcinogenesis [8, 9].

The use of kaolin, silver nitrate, oil of gomenoil, meouili oil, olive oil, sarious gases or killed bacteria has been largely abandoned because of the high percentage of recurrences [2].

Intrapleural tetracycline was first used by Rubinson and Bolooky [10] as a pleural sclerosing agent in patients with malignant effusion. Its use has been emphasized by Stephenson [5], but there is no certain confirmation that this method produces an effective pleurodesis. The recent introduction into surgical and endoscopic practice of biological glues such as hemostatics or sealants for bronchial fistulas has suggested the use of these materials for pleurodesis in pneumothorax. Experimental studies suggest that fibrin glue may cause an increase in the tensile strength of the visceral pleura, which thus impedes air leakage. However, in a clinical study of 35 patients, Hansen demonstrated that fibrin glue does not induce the formation of significant pleural adhesions or pleural thickening [11]. The major limitation of all these procedures is that none of these sclerosing agents can be used in treating the underlying lung lesions that produced the pneumothorax.

In 1989, we reported our initial experience in the use of the YAG-laser via pleuroscopy in 15 patients with spontaneous pneumothorax [12]. The YAG-laser is a very effective tool. Directed to the visceral pleura of the lung, it is able to coagulate and seal any blebs due to the aerostatic power of the YAG-laser on the pulmonary parenchyma. Subsequently, for the purpose of pleurodesis, the thermic effect of the laser directed at the parietal pleura is capable of producing an actual thermic pleurisy, the healing of which leads to adequate pleural adhesion.

2. Method

Since YAG-laser energy delivered to the parietal pleura is very painful, general anesthesia and deep

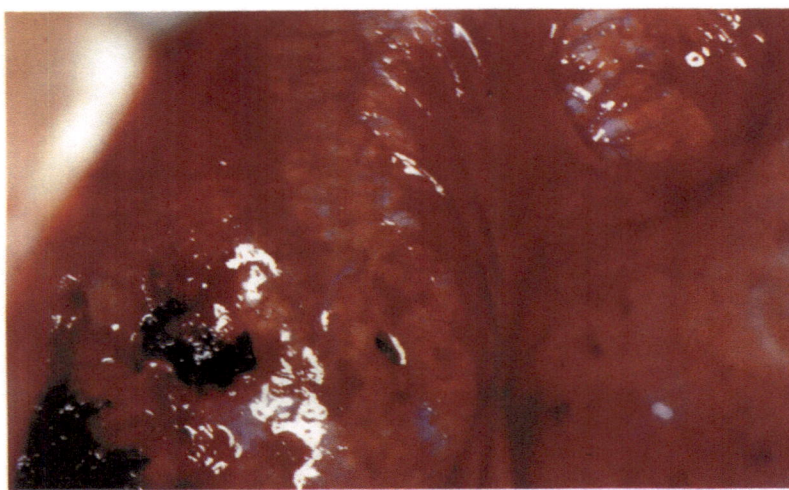

Fig. 44. Surgical view. Effect of YAG-laser pleurodesis

analgesia is mandatory. A double lumen tube is required to permit better exploration of the pleural cavity. The entire procedure is generally performed under one lung ventilation. A pulse oximeter must be used to monitor the patient.

The patient may be placed in a normal supine position or in lateral decubitus. Our first cases were treated with the patient positioned in normal supine decubitus and with the trocar inserted in the second intercostal space in the mid-clavicular line. This gives superb access to the lung apex but not for exploration of the lower lobe and is ineffective for pleurodesis of the lower part of the chest wall.

For this reason we soon adopted the position of lateral decubitus with the patient lying on the opposite side.

The trocar is inserted in the fourth intercostal space in the anterior axillary line. This access provides an excellent view of the apex of the chest cavity and of the lung apex and the dorsal parietal pleura is easily seen from the apex to the diaphragm.

In our experience only one trocar has been necessary for this treatment.

A 10 mm trocar must be inserted through a 1-2 cm incision. A telescope with a direct view is inserted as a first step in order to obtain a general view of the lung and of the pleural surface.

Any adhesions found must be freed with the YAG-laser to better explore all the lung parenchyma. If no blebs are discovered, 100-200 ml of sterile water can be introduced into the pleural cavity and the lung must be gently inflated in order to exclude any air leak from microscopic lesions. The first step of the procedure is pleural abrasion to obtain pleuro-

desis. The sterile fiber of the YAG-laser is introduced through the operative channel of a thoracoscope and directed to the parietal pleura. In order to avoid any risk of damage to the intercostal structures, the YAG-laser energy is directed to the parietal pleura covering the ribs (Fig. 44). Starting from the first rib in the dome of the chest, the parietal pleura covering the ribs is carbonized and coagulated to the maximum extent possible .

Usually, lines of pleurodesis extending for 15-20 cm can be easily produced. With the patient in lateral decubitus and the trocar inserted into the anterior axillary line, all the parietal pleura in the posterior chest wall may be easily abraded with the YAG-laser starting from the first to the eight rib. No pleurodesis is usually attempted on the diaphragm.

By changing the position of the operator and the direction of the fiber, the energy can be directed to the anterior part of the chest. With this access only a small part of the lateral parietal pleura remains unavailable for pleurodesis. A second incision in the parasternal area or posteriorly may be useful in completing the pleurodesis proved unnecessary in our experience. The energy delivered is largerly dependent on the quality of the fiber, the color of the zone and the distance from the point of irradiation. Usually we perform pleurodesis using continuous wave pulses of 30-50 w/s.

At the end of the pleurodesis the YAG-laser energy is directed to the lung surface and any blebs present can be easily sealed.

In order to better maintain the healing of the visceral pleura previously treated with the laser, we recently applied 5 ml of fibrin glue (Tissucol Immuno, Italy) through a double-channel catheter advanced through the second operative channel of the thoracoscope. After coagulation of the glue (5-6 min) the procedure can be concluded. Under direct visualisation the lung is gently inflated and a chest tube is positioned through the thoracoscope incision. If there is no air leak in the postoperative period, the chest tube can be removed 24-36 hours after the operation.

3. Results

Since 1986 more than 50 patients have been treated in our department with this procedure, without major complications. The average postoperative hospital stay was 4 days.

In two patients complete reexpansion of the lung was not achieved because of continuous air leak. These two patients presented at endoscopy multiple large bullae with a diameter of more than 3 cm. The YAG-laser directed to the bullae was ineffective in sealing the lung parenchyma and at thoracotomy a large hole in the lung apex was detected. These lesions were surgically resected and no further pleurodesis was considered desirable since the thermical pleurodesis inducted by the laser was considered sufficient. Two others patients were successfully treated and discharged from the hospital four and six days postoperatively. Thirty-five and 42 days later they developed recurrent pneumothorax in the lateral area of the chest X ray and were operated on. In both patients multiple small blebs were detected radiologically in the lower lobe, but not seen at endoscopy. In both patients the lung was solidly stuck to the parietal pleura in the anterior and posterior areas where the lines of pleurodesis were performed as evidence of the effectiveness of the YAG-laser pleurodesis.

In all the other patients the procedure was successful and no recurrences were found (maximum follow-up 60 months).

4. Discussion

The optimal treatment of patients with spontaneous pneumothorax remains a major cause of debate among thoracic surgeons. The knowledge that the cause inducing the pneumothorax is of little anatomic extent suggests that surgical operation is often disproportionate to the lesion as such.

Consequently, many authors have proposed the instillation into the pleural space of different substances capable of producing chemical or physical pleurodesis. Nevertheless, all these methods may produce various side-effects and the induction of permanent pleurodesis is uncertain.

For many years YAG-laser phototherapy has often been used by thoracic surgeons and chest physicians as a treatment for patients with endobronchial obstruction. This now has a well-established role in the palliation of advanced lung cancer [13]. In 1984 Wolfe and in 1985 LoCicero et al [14, 15] proposed the use of the YAG-laser for open lung resections, based on the YAG-laser's high cutting capability and especially the clinical and experimental evidence that both the YAG and CO_2 lasers could seal blood-vessels and small bronchi. Endoscopically, YAG-laser energy can be easily delivered through an operative thoracoscope. It can cut, burn, and coagulate simultaneously, so the risk of bleeding is minimal.

The rationale of any treatment in patients with spontaneous pneumothorax is to achieve the cure of the lung lesion and to produce an extensive and efficient pleurodesis. From this point of view, the YAG-laser can be considered a very effective tool.

Directed to the lung parenchyma, it is able to seal the air leak; directed to the parietal pleura it produces very good abrasion, thus inducing thermal pleurodesis. The cautery can also be useful in producing pleurodesis, but is less effective in sealing the air leak. In our experience the major limitation of the YAG-laser has been the impossibility of treating lung lesions greater than 3-4 cm. In such patients we believe that surgery remains mandatory.

In conclusion, given the need for ever less invasive therapeutic procedures, we consider that YAG-laser pleurodesis via thoracoscopy must be considered the therapy of choice in patients with spontaneous pneumothorax with the goal of definitive treatment.

References

1. Almind M, Lange P, Viskum K (1989) Spontaneous pneumothorax comparison of simple drainage, talc pleurodesis and tetracycline pleurodesis. Thorax 44 : 627-630
2. Singh SV (1979) Current status of parietal pleurectomy in recurrent pneumothorax. Scand J Thor Cardiovasc Surg 13 : 93-96
3. Spengler L (1906) Zur Chirurgie des Pneumothorax. Beitr Klin Chir 49 : 80
4. Bethune N (1935) Pleural poudrage. A new technique for the deliberate production of pleural adhesion as a preliminary to lobectomy. J Thorac Surg 4 : 251
5. Stephenson LW (1985) Treatment of pneumothorax with intrapleural tetracycline. Chest 88, 6 : 803-804

6. Daniel MT, Tribble CG, Rodgers BM (1990) Thoraco-scopy and talc poudrage for pneumothorax and effusion. Ann Thorac. Surg 50 : 186-189

7. Singer JJ, Jones YC, Tragermann LY (1941) Aseptic pleuritis experimentally produced. J Thorac Surg 10 : 251

8. Gaensler EA (1956) Parietal pleurectomy for recurrent spontaneous pneumothorax. Surg Gynecol Obstet 102 : 293

9. Jackon JW, Bennet MH (1973) Chest wall tumor following iodized talc pleurodesis. Thorax 28 : 788-793

10. Rubinson RM, Bolooky H (1972) Intrapleural tetracycline for control of malignant pleural effusion. A preliminary report. South Med J 65 : 847-849

11. Hansen MK, Kruse Andersen S, Boolsen Watt S, Andersen K (1989) Spontaneous pneumothorax and fibrin glue sealant during thoracoscopy. Eur J Cardio Thorac Surg 3 : 512-514

12. Torre M, Belloni PA (1989) Nd Yag laser pleurodesis through thoracoscopy: new curative therapy in spontaneous pneumothorax. Ann Thor Surg 47 : 887-889

13. Torre M, Barbieri B, Donatelli F, Ravini M, Rizzato GF, Belloni PA (1987) Unusual endobronchial extension of lung tumor treated with YAG-laser and surgery. Thorax 42 : 899-990

14. Wolfe WG, Cole PH, Sabiston DC (1984) Experimental and clinical use of the Nd YAG-laser in the management of pulmonary neoplasm. Ann Surg 199 : 526-531

15. LoCicero J, Hartz RS, Frederiksen JW, Micaelis LC (1985) New applications of the laser in the pulmonary surgery. Hemostasis and sealing of air leaks. Ann Thor Surg 40 : 546-550

Thoracoscopic treatment of pneumothorax
Pleural abrasion and pleurectomy

J.F. Levi and Ph. Kleinmann

1. Introduction

Parietal pleurectomy and surgical pleural abrasion are the best preventive treatments for recurrent pneumothorax. Classically, their performance necessitates thoracotomy. The incidence of postoperative pain, muscular, functional and esthetic sequelae has led to development of a percutaneous technique of parietal pleurectomy and pleural abrasion avoiding thoracotomy [1]. Medical pleurodesis techniques have been in use for many years. They all rely on intrapleural administration of a substance that irritates the pleura. All of these techniques are less effective since the risk of pneumothorax recurrence remains high, from 7% to 20% according to various authors. Talc pleurodesis [2, 3], the most effective medical procedure, presents disadvantages which are not negligible: recurrence in 5% to 13% of cases; risk of suppuration; risk of foreign body reaction if intraparenchymal passage of talc occurs; postoperative pain; and transitory fever.

Therefore the best prevention of spontaneous pneumothorax recurrence seemed to consist of open thoracic surgical procedures, namely pleural abrasion and pleurectomy. The rates of recurrence are respectively less than 2% and 1% for these two surgical techniques for which the mortality is zero in idiopathic spontaneous pneumothorax [4, 8]. However, these surgical procedures have a high morbidity, evaluated at from 5% to 10% with severe complications occurring in two-thirds [9]. The occurrence of hemothorax, which necessitates reoperation in 1% to 2% of cases, notably increases the risk of requiring a blood transfusion [6, 9]. For these reasons, some authors have modified the procedures in order to decrease morbidity. The surgical approach was changed by using axillary incisions [8] and incisions in the nonmuscular triangle [10, 11], and apical pleurectomies [7] were performed instead of subtotal classical pleurectomies [12]. It seemed a logical consequence, using thoracic video-surgery, to perform pleurectomies and pleural abrasions without thoracotomy in order to eliminate entirely the morbidity linked to thoracotomy.

2. Operative technique

Endoscopic surgery of the thorax permits carrying out the same operations as in open thorax conditions, but without requiring thoracotomy, by use of instrumental procedures through the different entry sites.

Operative conditions necessary for endoscopic thoracic surgery are the same as for classical surgery. The operation is performed in the operating room on a patient under general anesthesia with cardiac and oxymetric monitoring.

Selective intubation is necessary and the patient is placed in the postero-lateral thoracotomy position (Fig. 45) with the arm on side the operation resting free in a protected padded armrest.

The surgeon and his assistant operate from the back of the patient while the medical instrument technician is in front of them, with the video cart placed before the patient, at his head.

The choice between pleural abrasion or pleurectomy varies according to authors. Although no prospective studies have compared the efficacity of these two techniques, they seem to be equally effective according to different series in the literature [4, 8]. However, pleural abrasion offers the principal advantages of its technical simplicity, shorter opera-

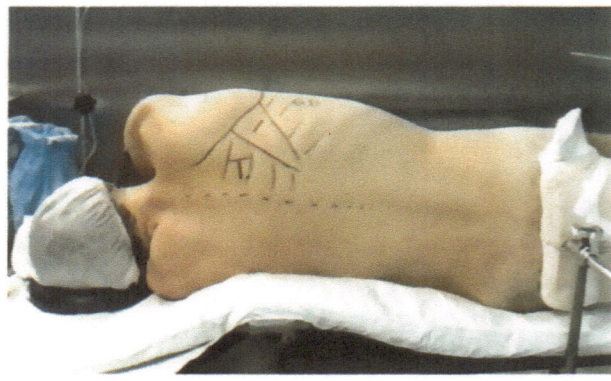

Fig. 45. Patient placed in the postero-lateral thoracotomy position ; the black line represents the posterior orifice in the non-muscular area beetween trapezius (T) and latissimus dorsi (GD)

tion time, and especially the possiblility of thoracic reoperation, which cannot be excluded in young heavy smokers and in those who are potential transplantation patients. Such reoperation is possible since the extrapleural layer has been preserved. Insofar as pleurectomy is concerned, it makes impossible simple dissection in the extrapleural plane and considerably increases the difficulty of repeated surgical operation as well as its hemorrhagic risk. In case of previous pleurectomy, extracorporeal circulation is formally contraindicated [13]. Despite these disadvantages, pleurectomy is still considered the best choice by some authors.

Regardless of the endoscopic pleurodesis technique used, careful exploration of the lung is necessary, with parenchymal resection if bullous lesions exist.

2.1. Pleural abrasion under thoracic video-surgery

The first 10 mm trocar, used for introduction of the camera optical system, is inserted in the posterior nonmuscular area. One must be careful to insert it low enough (6th intercostal space) so as not to be hindered by overhanging of the upper adjacent ribs. Even more caution is required in thin or female patients whose intercostal spaces are narrow. If the immediate preoperative film confirms presence of a pneumothorax, the second trocar can be directly introduced with the habitual precautions of installing a thoracic drain. If the pneumothorax has been resorbed at the time of operation, there exists a risk of pulmonary injury at introduction of the trocar. Under these circumstances, after cutaneous incision with a scalpel, it is preferable to spread apart the intercostal

muscles, then open the parietal pleura under visual control with soft-tipped forceps. This permits reestablishment of the pneumothorax and safe trocar placement. A second 5 mm trocar is introduced under endoscopic surveillance. Its insertion is made on the anterior axillary line in the 3rd or 4th space (Fig. 45). This opening must be anterior enough to permit good exposure of pulmonary lesions. Through this trocar a pulmonary retractor is introduced. Concerning pleural abrasion, the first operative step always consists of treatment of parenchymal lesions. It begins with freeing of the parietal adhesions present (Figs. 46, 47), then treatment of bullous lesions (Fig. 48). These different steps will be covered in detail in the next chapter. Stapling with the endoscopic stapling device of dystrophic bullous lesions necessitates placement of a 3rd trocar 12 mm in diameter. It is introduced under video control on the mid-axillary line in the 7th intercostal space. Its position must be anterior enough to allow for a good orientation of the forceps in the intercostal space axis towards the apex, especially in thin patients. Once pulmonary lesions have been treated, mechanical pleural abrasion is carried out. This is performed using a pleural brush (Fig. 49) which is doubly curved thus allowing access to all areas of the thoracic cavity. In the first step, it is introduced through the 12 mm trocar opening, with video monitoring made possible by introduction of the endoscopic telescope through the 10 mm posterior trocar. The curvature of the brush prevents its introduction through a trocar. Airtightness of the chest wall is unnecessary during the operation, since selective intubation with ventilation of one lung is used. This instrument permits mechanical abrasion from the apex to the costodiaphragmatic recess. In order to perform abrasion of the anterior surfaces, the entry sites for the telescope and the brush are inverted. Abrasion must be continued until development of a uniform hemorrhagic dotting (Fig. 50). Once the abrasion has been performed, two 20 F drains are put into place, one through the superior axillary opening oriented towards the apex, and the other through the inferior axillary opening oriented towards the base. After abrasion of the diaphragmatic pleura 40 cc of 30% glucose solution are instilled into the inferior drain. At the time of reexpansion it is essential to check proper position of the upper drain.

2.2. Percutaneous parietal pleurectomy

This involves a pleurectomy technique performed under video control concerning the parietal pleura. This method permits carrying out a subtotal pleurectomy and notably facilitates its performance in the

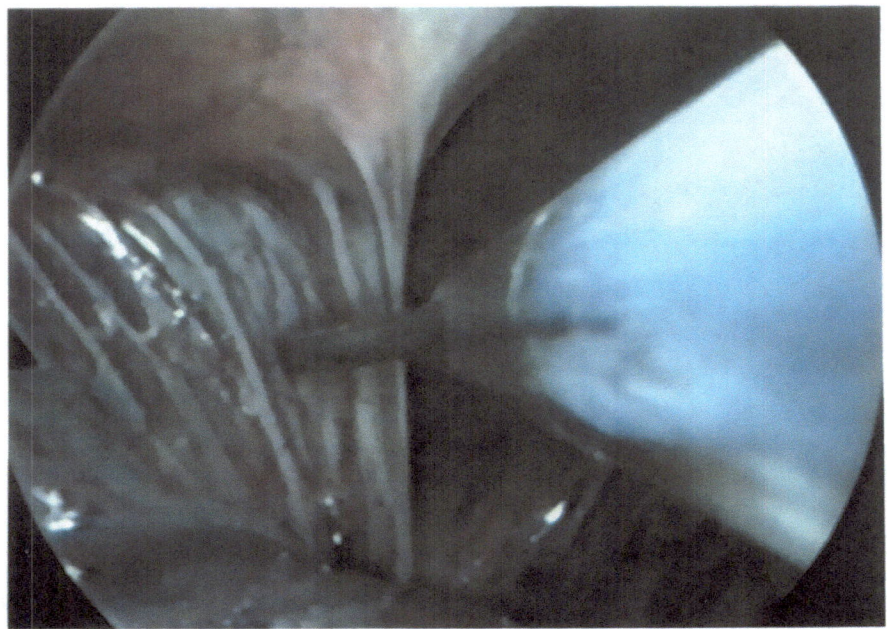

Fig. 46. Pleuro-parenchymal adhesion divided by endoscopic scissors introduced through the optic's channel

Fig. 47. Short pleuro-parenchymal adhesion sectioned by scissors introduced through another 5 mm canula

Fig. 48. Endoscopic view of an apical bulla (2 cm diameter)

46

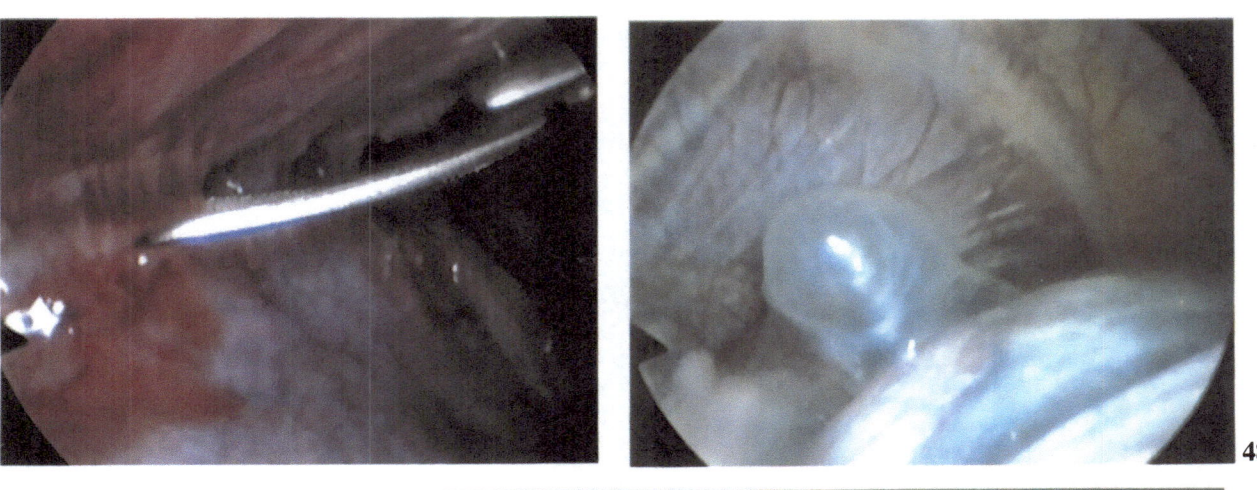

47

48

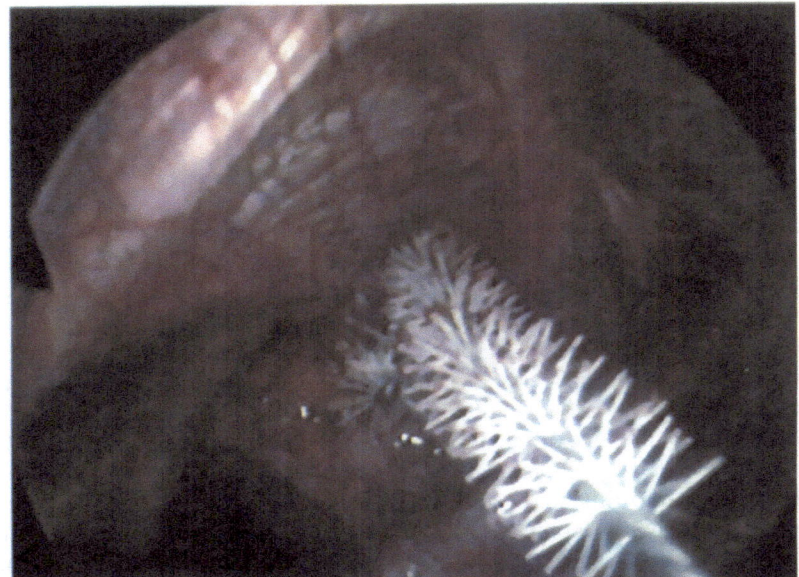

Fig. 49. Double-curved pleural brush performing abrasive pleurodesis

49

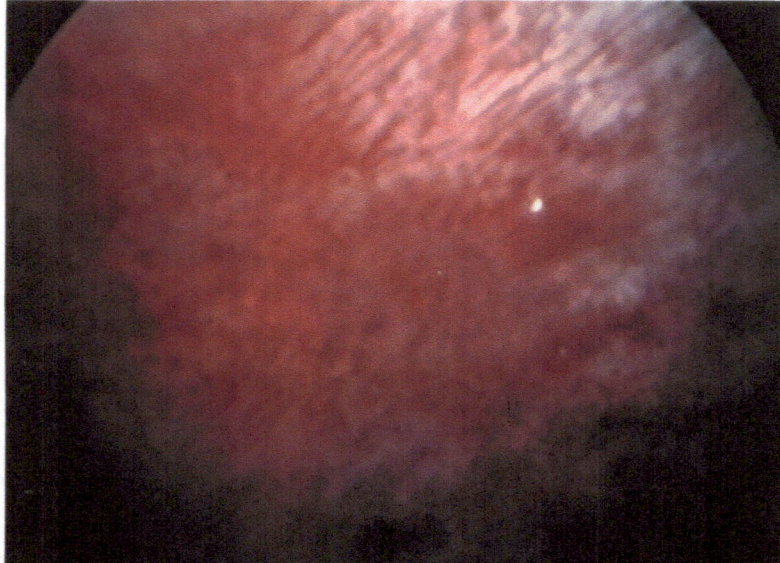

Fig. 50. Uniform hemorrhagic dotting of the parietal pleura

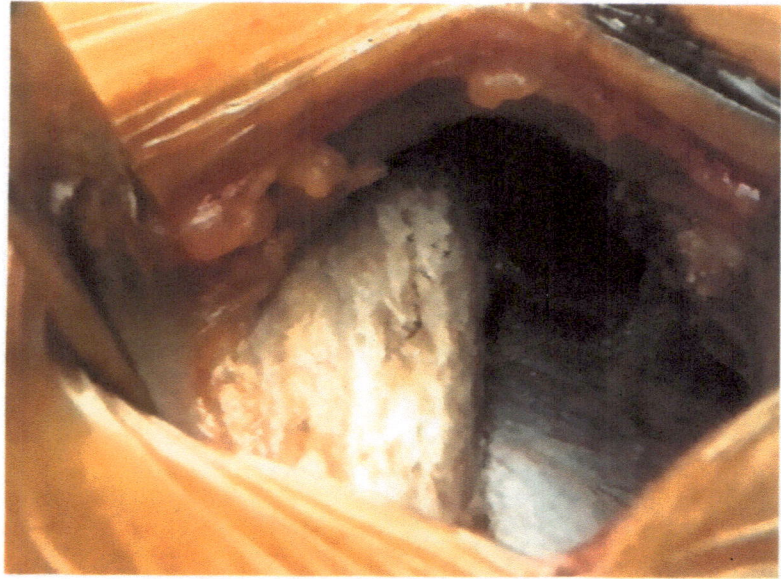

Fig. 51. Parietal-pleura is approached by disinsertion of the intercostal muscle at the upper edge of the sixth rib over 2 to 3 cm

anterior areas where the pleura is thin and adheres very closely to the thoracic wall. The operation begins with a 3 cm incision in the nonmuscular triangle posteriorly (an area of lesser pleural adherence) (Fig. 45). The extrapleural plane is approached by disinsertion of the intercostal muscle at the upper edge of the sixth rib over 2 to 3 cm (Fig. 51). The detachment of the extrapleural layer is begun using small dry gauze compresse. The endoscope is next introduced into this space and the detachment continued under video control. This detachment is pursued using small gauze compresses held by long forceps introduced parallel to the endoscope (Fig. 52).

In difficult areas, especially the anterior part of the thorax, this detachment may be pursued using scissors introduced through the operating channel of the endoscope (Fig. 53). This technique permits a perfect anatomic bloodless detachment which preserves the parietal vascular pedicles. Detachment extends as follows: superiorly, to the external arch of the 1st rib; anteriorly, to 1.5 cm in front of the internal mammary vessels; posteriorly, to the costovertebral recess (Fig. 54) but somewhat remote from the sympathetic nerve; and inferiorly, to a horizontal line along the middle arch of the 9th rib (Fig. 55), performing a genuine subtotal pleurectomy. Once the detachment

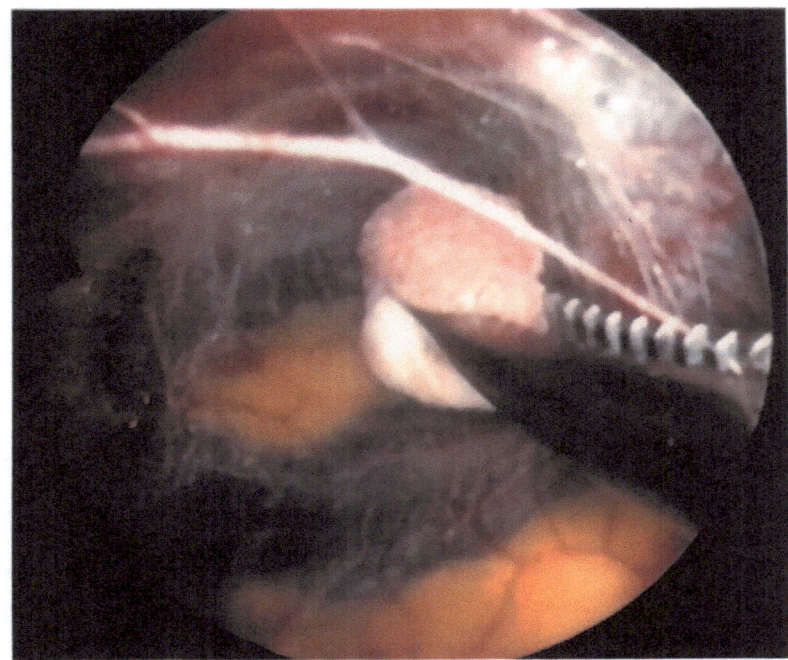

Fig. 52. The extrapleural detachment is pursued using small gauze compresse held by long forceps introduced parallel to the endoscope

52

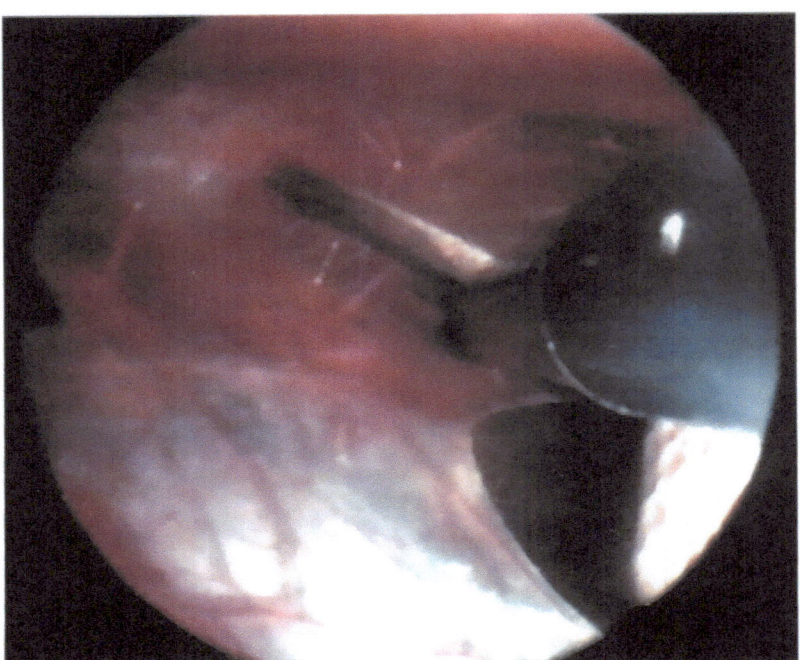

Fig. 53. The extrapleural detachment is pursued using scissors introduced through the operating channel of the endoscope, note a hole in the thin fragile parietal pleura below the scissors

53

is done, a second axillary trocar is inserted. The latter permits endopleural control of the pleurectomy and facilitates pleural sectioning. This sectioning is carried out with scissors after electrocoagulation (Fig. 56) or blade coagulation of the pleura. Section-coagulation must be done at least 1.5 cm away from the thoracic wall in order to avoid diffusion effects of electrocautery and lesions of the intercostal nerves. Once the pleurectomy is finished, exploration

and treatment of parenchymal lesions as previously described is done.

2.3. Intrapleural pleurectomy

This involves an exclusively intrapleural pleurectomy technique which only allows performance of apical pleurectomy. Two (axillary and posterior) trocars as

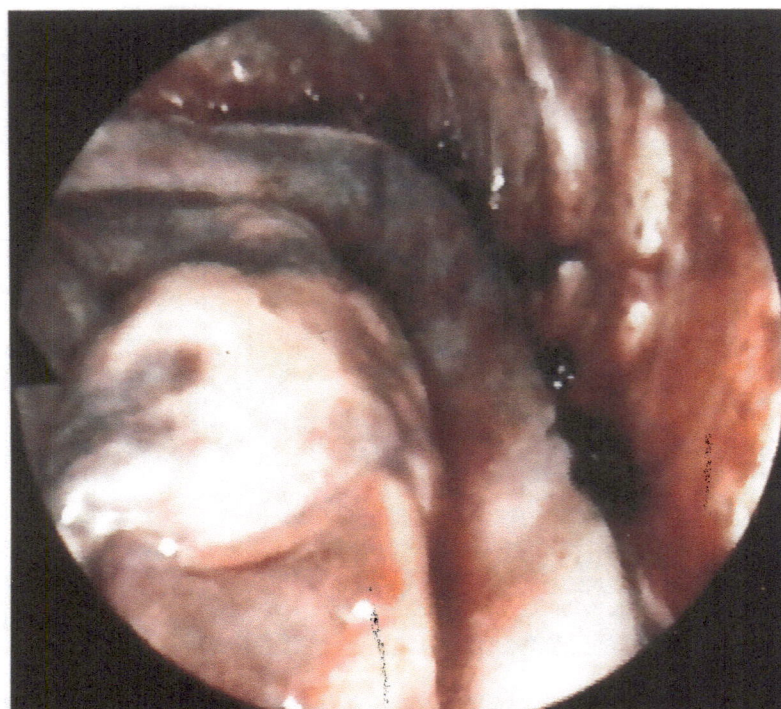

54

Fig. 54. Apical and posterior boundaries of the parietal pleurectomy. On the right is the costo-vertebral recess, the apex in at the top of the figure

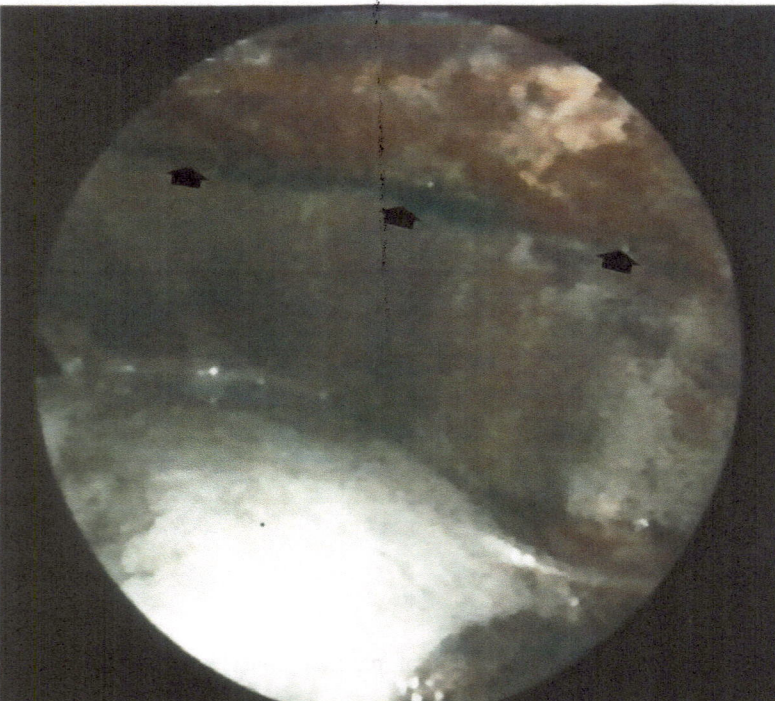

55

Fig. 55. The interior limit *(arrows)* of the parietal pleurectomy is a horizontal line along the middle arch of the 9th rib. The diaphragm is at the lower part of the photograph

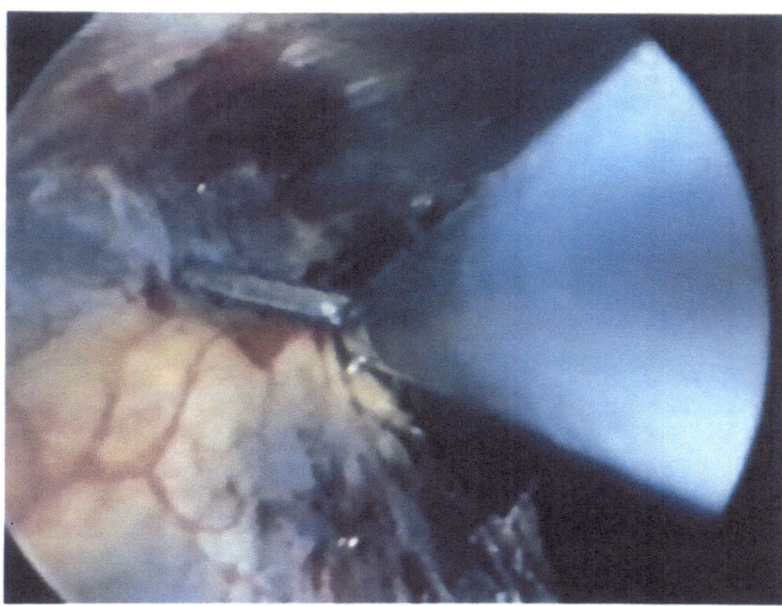

Fig. 56. Pleural section with electrocoagulating scissors

previously described are needed. The limits of the pleurectomy are demarcated by electrocoagulation of the parietal pleura using an electrode spatula. These limits are as follows: superiorly, the external arch of the 1st rib; anteriorly, 1.5 cm in front of the internal mammary vessels; posteriorly, the costovertebral recess; and inferiorly, by a horizontal line along the middle arch of the 5th rib. Once the outer limits of the pleurectomy have been designated, the area of pleurectomy is separated into a series of parallel strips (Fig. 57). The strips of pleura thus delimited are resected by simple traction using forceps and freed using scissors (Fig. 58). In this technique, exploration and treatment of bullous lesions precedes the pleurodesis.

3. Results

From August 1990 to April 1992, 120 patients were treated using video-surgery for spontaneous pneumothorax. These were cases of recurrent spontaneous pneumothorax among which 23 were bilateral cases and 11 were air leakage lasting over 10 days old. 68 patients were treated by percutaneous parietal pleurectomy and 52 by percutaneous pleural abrasion. The technical performance of the operation was possible in all cases.

The operative blood loss was 40 cc +/-10 cc versus 250 cc after classical thoracotomy. No patient was transfused during or after surgery. The average operating time for percutaneous parietal pleurectomy was 90 minutes and for pleural abrasion 45 minutes. Duration of drainage had a mean value of 4 days (extreme values: 2-28 days). No postoperative hemothorax occurred. One patient presented a thoracic wall abscess arising from a subjacent pneumopathy. Six patients presented prolonged postoperative air leaks (>14 days). Ten patients who were treated by parietal pleurectomy without apical resection using stapling technique on bullous lesions (i.e. before the advent of endoscopic staplers) presented a postoperative air effusion forming a pouch above the diaphragm necessitating further drainage in the 3 weeks following surgery. One patient treated by endoscopic pleural abrasion presented a postoperative apical pouch with spontaneous resolution without drainage. Another patient presented a postoperative air effusion treated by drainage one month after endoscopic pleural abrasion.

The mean hospitaliation was 6 days (extreme values : 4-30 days) versus 10 days after classical surgery.

Patients did not suffer from immediate postoperative pain as in thoracotomy. They only complained about the drains. Postoperative pain was three times less severe, as evaluated by the Analog Visual Scale (see Table 1) [14, 15], than in classical open surgery [4]. At the 5th day patient self-evaluation for pain reached 0.

FEV1 measured at 2 months postoperatively was found to be on the average 92% of theoretical normal FEV1 levels (extreme values: 59% - 118%). This demonstrates the absence of adverse respiratory consequences of endoscopic thoracic surgery.

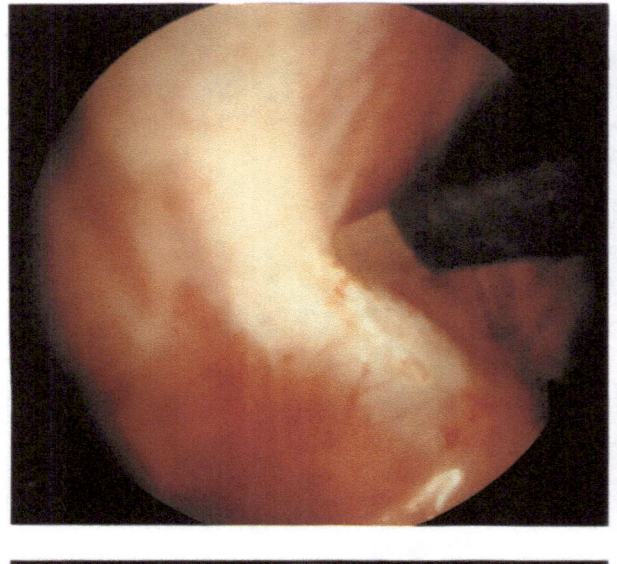

57a

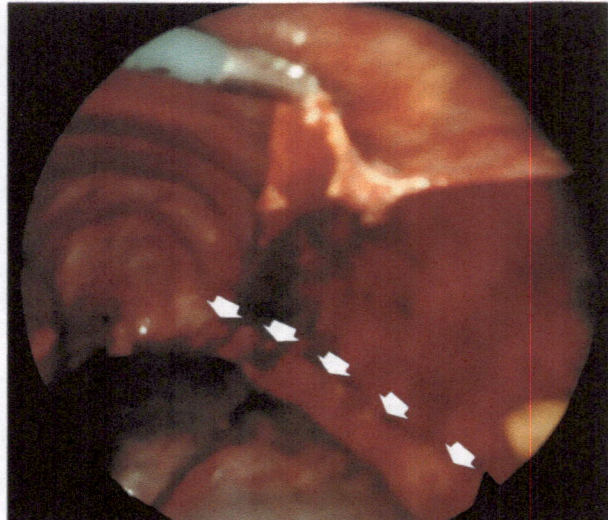

58

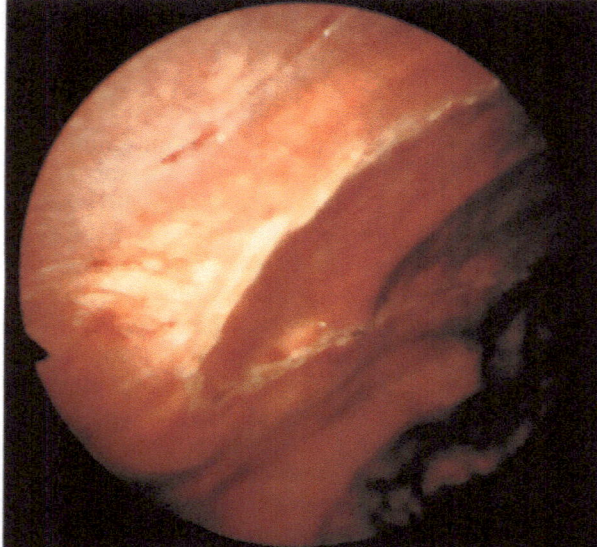

b

Fig. 57a-b. Technique of intrapleural pleurectomy :
a Pleural incision along the rib using electrode spatula.
b Design of a pleural flap

Fig. 58. Stripping of a pleural flap using forceps and scissors. *Arrows* indicate the posterior limits of the flap. (Photographs : D. Gossot)

Table 1. Immediate postoperative pain after percutaneous parietal pleurectomy and thoracotomy

Post op. day	D0	D1	D3	D4	D5
P.P.P.*	1.5	0.7	0.5	0.2	0
Thoracotomy	> 6.5			6.4	4.5

* P.P.P. = percutaneous parietal pleurectomy.
Postoperative pain evaluated by the Analogic Visual Scale (AVS) is scaled from 0 to 10.

No postoperative pulmonary complication occurred. Shoulder mobility was perfect on patient reawakening. Long-term postoperative recurrence has not occurred (>3 months).

4. Discussion

Parietal pleurectomy or pleural abrasion by endoscopic thoracic surgery avoids the disadvantages of thoracotomy while offering an identical procedure with regard to surgical pleurodesis techniques.

Exploration and resection of bullous lesions (blebs, dystrophy) are always combined with endoscopic pleurodesis.

Pleural abrasion and parietal pleurectomy, whose mortality levels are zero in idiopathic pneumothorax, have rates of recurrence of pneumothorax which are less than 1% [1, 2, 6].

In cases of synchronous bilateral pneumothorax a bilateral endoscopic pleurodesis is possible, thus avoiding classical sternotomy.

The advantages of endoscopic thoracic surgery over classical surgery are numerous. These advantages are all due to the fact that the disabling approach of thoracotomy is avoided:

— absence of thoracic wall muscular section and spreading of the intercostal space explains the major decrease in postoperative pain and absence of muscular sequelae;

— absence of adverse postoperative respiratory consequences permits resort to this method in pathologic contexts other than spontaneous idiopathic pneumothorax;

— constant surveillance of hemostasis limits bleeding during and after surgery;

— an esthetic advantage is evident as well as a reduction in duration of hospitalization.

For these reasons, thoracotomy no longer seems necessary for the effective treatment of recurrent spontaneous pneumothorax.

References

1. Levi JF, Kleinmann P, Riquet M, Debesse B (1990) Percutaneous parietal pleurectomy for recurrent spontaneous pneumothorax. Lancet 336 : 1577-1578
2. Guérin JC, Champel F, Biron E, Kalb JC (1985) Talcage pleural par thoracoscopie dans le traitement du pneumothorax. Rev Mal Resp 2 : 25-29
3. Weissberg D (1986) The Surgical Management of Recurrent Pneumothorax: Pleuroscopy and Talc Poudrage. In Kittle CF (ed.) Current Controversies in Thoracic Surgery. WB Saunders Philadelphia, pp. 46-50
4. Getz S, Beasley W (1983) Spontaneous pneumothorax. Am J Surg 145 : 823-827
5. Hansen AK et al (1989) Operative pleurodesis in spontaneous pneumothorax. Scand J Thor Cardiovasc Surg 23 : 279-281
6. Thomeret G, Debesse B, Reimund P, Elhadad A, Grenier G, Latarjet I (1976) La pleurectomie pariétale dans le traitement du pneumothorax idiopathique bénin. A propos de 101 pleurectomies chez 90 malades. Ann Chir Thorac. Card vasc 15 (2) 161-166
7. Weeden D, Smith GH (1983) Surgical experience in the management of spontaneous pneumothorax. Thorax 38 : 737-743
8. Deslauriers J, Beaulieu M, Despres JP et al (1980) Transaxillary pleurectomy for treatment of spontaneous pneumothorax. Ann Thorac Surg 30 : 569-574
9. Bojar R, Kittle CF (1986) The surgical management of recurrent or persistent pneumothorax: Pleurectomy. In Kittle CF (ed.) Current Controversies in Thoracic Surgery. WB Saunders Philadelphia pp. 51-57
10. Lau OJ, Shawkat S (1982) Pleurectomy through the triangle of auscultation. Thorax 37 : 945-946
11. Nazarian J, Down G, Lau OJ (1988) Pleurectomy through the triangle of auscultation for treatment of recurrent pneumothorax in younger patients. Arch Surg 123 : 113-114
12. Gaensler EA (1956) Parietal pleurectomy for recurrent pneumothorax. Surg Gynecol Obstet 102 : 293-308
13. Bonnette P, Bisson A, Ben el Kadi N, Colchen A, Leroy M, Caubarrere I, Fischler M, Loirat P (1990) Greffe Bipulmonaire. La double unipulmonaire
14. Wallenstein SL (1984) Measurement of pain and analgesia in cancer patients. Cancer 53 : 2360-2366
15. Marin I, Lepresle C, Mechet MA, Debesse B (1991) Douleur postopératoire au décours d'une thoracotomie, étude de 116 malades. Rev Fr Mal Resp 8 : 213-216

Endoscopic procedures in lung and mediastinal surgery

Ph. Kleinmann and J.F. Levi

1. Introduction

The perfection of endoscopic thoracic surgical techniques with regard to pneumothorax [4, 5] has logically led to treatment of the lung parenchyma . Initially, the lung was explored and treated only in cases of pedicular bullous lesions by a loop technique [4-6] or for simple lung biopsies (for diagnostic purposes) which were always risky [1, 3]. Laser destruction of blebs or bullous lesions (Fig. 59) of the lung was performed later by others [7, 8].

The development of endoscopic surgical instruments and the advent of endoscopic staplers have permitted performance of true lung parenchymal resection and consequently broadened the indications for endoscopic thoracic surgery.

This chapter is intended to describe the technical conditions required in the performance of endoscopic thoracic surgery, then to concisely explain the particular techniques applied to the different pulmonary pathologic entities.

2. Common techniques and equipment used in endoscopic thoracic surgery

2.1. Equipment

The equipment used in endoscopic surgery has already been described in another chapter. The instruments more specifically used for lung resection are as follows:

– a non-traumatic lung retractor which permits exploration and perfect exposure of the lesions to be excised;

– prehensile ratchet forceps which must be non-traumatic (i.e. without claws) to help in the manipulations;

– short forceps (35 cm) and long forceps (45 cm);

– a set of straight and curved forceps;

– and the endoscopic stapler without which this surgery would not have come about.

Regardless of whether 3 or 6 cm rows of staples are applied, certain technical conditions must be met for the use of the stapler. The length of these instruments (45 cm) requires that the operative opening be not too close to the lesions to be resected. The two jaws of the instrument must always be visible. These endoscopic staplers necessitate placement of a 12 mm or 18 mm trocar for their introduction.

2.2. Technique

The operation is carried out in the operating room, the patient under general anesthesia with selective intubation. The patient is installed in the lateral thoracotomy position. Only in this position can the entire lung be explored and access obtained to the mediastinum and diaphragm. The patient's arm is dependent or put into an elevated cradle if a trocar is to be placed in the axilla. A cushion is needed to protect the shoulder, enlarging the operative field including the operative openings of the axilla above the hip and the shoulder. The operative field is large enough to allow true thoracotomy if necessary. The monitoring systems are at the head of the patient while the surgeon is situated at the patient's back. Insufflation is most often not required.

Under certain circumstances the patient is put in the supine position:

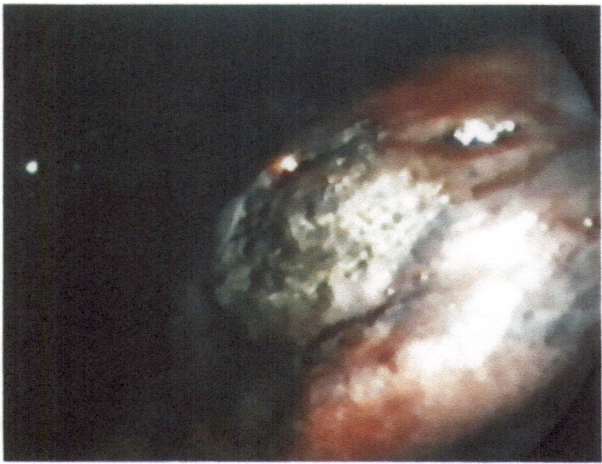

Fig. 59. Bulla laserisation with a CO_2 laser

– for surgery of the pericardium if a voluminous effusion exists;

– and the presence of respiratory insufficiency contraindicating both selective intubation and the thoracotomy position.

2.3. Surgical approaches

Three incisions are usually required in order to perform a resection of lung parenchyma. One opening is almost always constant: the posterior opening.

The posterior opening is made behind the caudal tip of the scapula in the non-muscular zone between the anterior edge of the trapezius, the spinal edge of the latissimus dorsi and the spinal border of the scapula (i.e. the triangle of auscultation). From this opening a thoracotomy may be performed if necessary. The incision is located in the 6th intercostal space (Fig. 60). If operative difficulties arise, the opening for the initial trocar may be transformed into a 2 to 3 cm incision, as when visual localisation of a parenchymal nodule is difficult or if the tissue to be excised is bulky.

Two other trocars are inserted, one with a 12 or 18 mm diameter (for the endostapler) and the other with a diameter of 5 or 10 mm. Their location depends on the site of the lesions to be resected. Most often they will be made on the anterior and mid-axillary lines from the 5th to the 8th intercostal spaces (Fig. 60). The three openings must always form a triangle whose apex is at the point furthest away from the lesions to be treated (12 mm trocar), and whose base is directly above or slightly behind the lesions (Fig. 61). The functions of these ports are of course interchangeable during surgery.

2.4. Beginning the operation

The operation always begins with an approach to the pleural cavity and creation of a pneumothorax.

Through the posterior opening, the endothoracic fascia is reached by retraction of the intercostal muscle fibers with a blunt tip forceps. The parietal pleura is opened creating a pneumothorax under visual control. This step is only necessary in the absence of either pneumothorax or abundant pleural effusion (i.e. the lung and the parietal pleura are in contact with each other). For these reasons a routine chest x-ray film is always made before surgery. The direct route into the pleural cavity is preferred rather than blind penetration of a trocar, whether or not the trocar has a smooth tip or is equipped with a safety device, since its tip can injure the lung parenchyma. The risk of parenchymal lesions occurring upon entry of the trocar is considerable if pleuroparenchymal adhesions exist. Consequently, all medical history of pleural disease, infection or drainage calls for caution and therefore installation of the first trocar under visual surveillance. The other trocars are introduced under endoscopic surveillance after the first exploration .

The installation of the endopleural fiberoptic instrument permits an initial exploration, checking on the pneumothorax and searching for pleuro-parenchymal adhesions (Fig. 62) which are carefully divided.

This division is carried out using electrocoagulation scissors or by a surgical blade (Fig. 63) introduced through the operating channel of the optical device. The latter is very useful during this step especially if adhesions are numerous (Fig. 64). A suction device is placed via another entry site for removal of smoke and for stretching tissues to be divided. Pleurolysis is an essential step. Completion of debridement of the peripheral surface of the lung is evident since residual adhesions will mask the pleural cavity. It is also necessary to perfectly debride the mediastinal surface of the lung. These steps facilitate mobilization of the lung. Section of the pulmonary ligament is required if surgery on the basal pyramid is intended. Exploration leads to accurate determination of the topography of the lesions and precise positioning of the other ports.

2.5. Drainage

Two drains are inserted via the anterior and middle axillary openings, one at apical level and the other at the base. Usually, small drains are used (18 F), but if the pleura is inflammatory or the parenchyma dystrophic, one of the drains is larger (28 F).

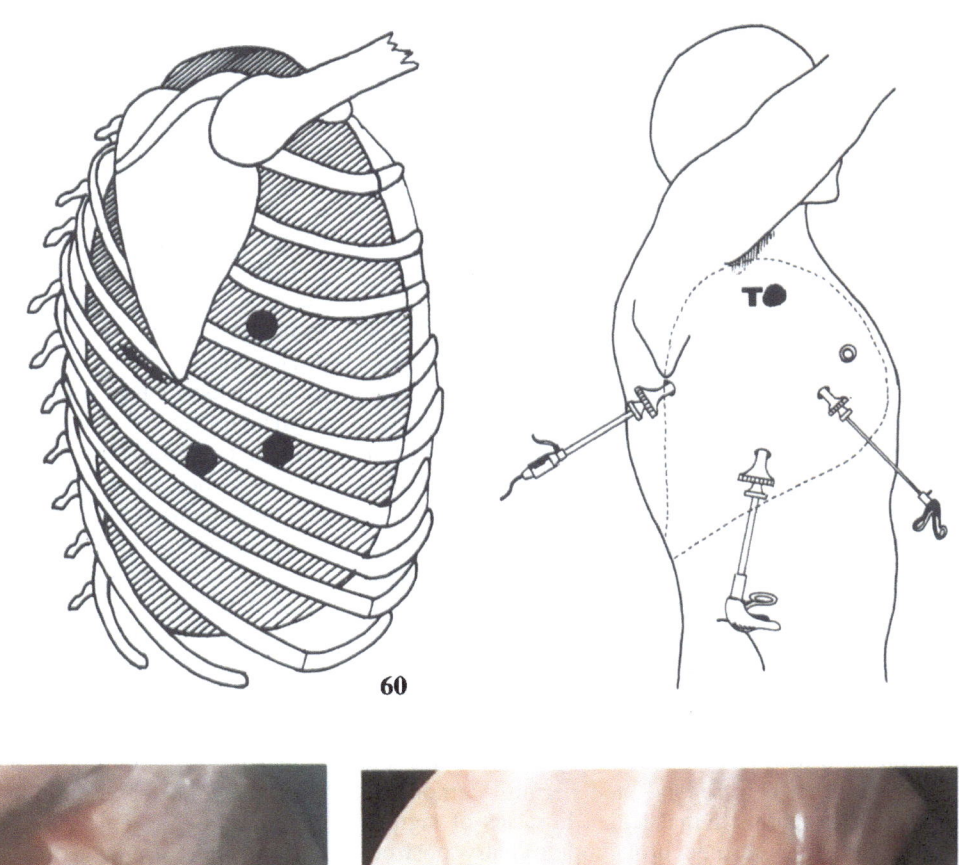

Fig. 60. Operative sites for trocars, the posterior site is represented by an arrow

Fig. 61. Three openings forming a triangle whose apex (12 mm trocar for stapler) is at the point furthest away from the lesion to be treated, here an apical tumor (T)

60

61

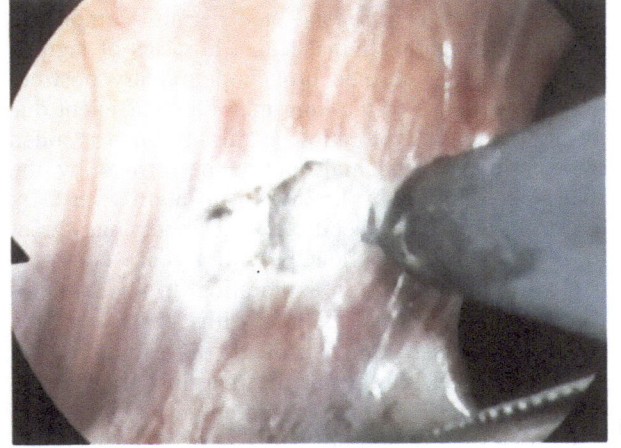

62

63

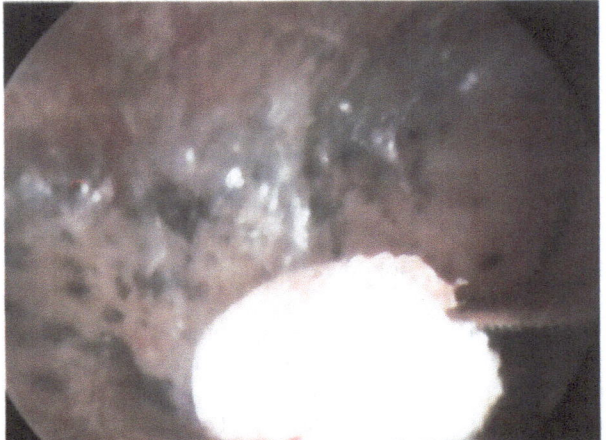

Fig. 62. Thin pleuro-parenchymal adhesion

Fig. 63. Wide pleuro-parenchymal adhesion severed by a coagulating blade

Fig. 64. Total adhesion between lung and parietal pleura, pleurolysis is done here by a dry gauze compress (< 1 cm)

64

3. Resection of lung parenchyma

The particular operative aspects of resection of lung parenchyma with respect to the various pneumological conditions will be discussed in the next three sections.

3.1. Pulmonary resection and pneumothorax

Resection of parenchyma is an integral part of the surgical treatment of spontaneous recurrent pneumothorax by endoscopic thoracic surgery. Whether carried out in the context of an endoscopic parietal pleurectomy (EPP) or an endoscopic pleural abrasion (EPA), after debridement and performance of the pleural stage, the treatment of the parenchyma begins by careful exploration.

This necessitates perfect coordination between the surgeon and the anesthesiologist, the latter checking the reexpansion of the lung on the monitor. A too abrupt ventilation results in excessive reexpansion and obscuring of the visual field by the ventilated lung. The exploration is carried out in two steps, first in the free pleural cavity, and then after instillation of from 150 to 250 cc of physiologic saline into the pleural cavity. This second step permits demonstration of pleuroparenchymal leaks. In cases of significant preexisting chronic bronchopulmonary obstruction, the collapse of the lung may be insufficient due to air trapping. Exploration in this instance is aided by continuous bronchial suction performed by the anesthesiologist or by limited insufflation with CO_2. The utilisation of a specific lung parenchyma retractor or tripodal forceps loaded with a gauze compress is always very helpful in exploration. In this pathologic context, one must explore with special care the apical and dorsal segments of the superior lobe, the segment of Nelson and all the margins. Exploration may be negative, but most often either pedicular bullous lesions are found (Figs. 65, 66), or blebs (Fig. 67), or networks of bullous lesions more or less well spread out (Fig. 68), or more exceptionally a pleuropulmonary fistula (Fig. 69).

Apical resection is performed through three openings forming a triangle with an axillary base (Fig. 61). The posterior opening already described is consistently made. The anterior opening is made along the anterior axillary line; it must be low enough to allow introduction of long instruments and for the surgeon not to be hindered by the patient's shoulder.

The third opening is located on the mid-axillary line at the level of the 7th or 8th intercostal space. It must not be too low, especially in women, in order not to be obstructed by the hip. These two openings usually serve as optic passages or for introduction of the endoscopic stapler.

After localising the lesions to be resected, nontraumatic ratchet forceps are introduced via the anterior opening to expose the lesions. The presentation of lesions may be improved by using forceps with a longer grip (digestive clamp type) placed below the future resection zone. Then, according to the line of resection desired, the stapler is introduced via one of the other openings. The stapler must only be applied to healthy parenchyma. The two jaws of the stapling device must be checked before suturing and sectioning. In fact, since application of the stapler is performed on an excluded lung, it is imperative to be sure that no segments of parenchyma normally distant from one another be stapled together: the resultant pulmonary fold would cause a major deficit in reexpansion and ventilation.

Several applications of the stapler are necessary to effectuate an adequate apical resection, i.e. from three to six 30 mm rows are most often used; however, fewer rows of 60 mm length may be used. The successive applications of the stapler must not leave spaces of healthy parenchyma between the rows.

In case of voluminous bullous lesions (> 10 cm) (Figs. 70, 71), the technique is quite identical. Tight adhesions beetween bullae, chest wall and mediastinum are very frequent and must be totally eliminated. This step must be done very carefully in order to avoid injuring adjacent structures such as the phrenic nerve, superior vena cava or azygos vein. Complete freeing of the bullae is essential in order to locate their base of implantation. The exposure is facilitated by opening of the bullous lesion (Fig. 72) and its collapse (Fig. 73) effected either by electrocoagulation scissors or laser. Next, the internal surface of the bullous lesion is checked for air leakage. Endobullous debridement is performed by electrocoagulation. Localisation of the base of bullous implantation (Fig. 74) is essential in order to apply the stapler effectively (Fig. 75). It is even more important here than in cases of spontaneous pneumothorax since the parenchyma is emphysematous and air leaks after resection frequently occur in this dystrophic parenchyma. If the bullous base is irregular or very large, the bulla is gradually resected from one end of its base towards the other (the importance of the laser in this step is considerable), then the verges are mechanically or manually sutured together after apposition. Since the lung is often wholly dystrophic it is useful to measure the thickness of the parenchyma in order to correctly choose the appropriate staples in each case. A diffuse emphysematous dystrophy and proximity of the pulmonary vasculature are the main obstacles to the endoscopic excision of giant bullae.

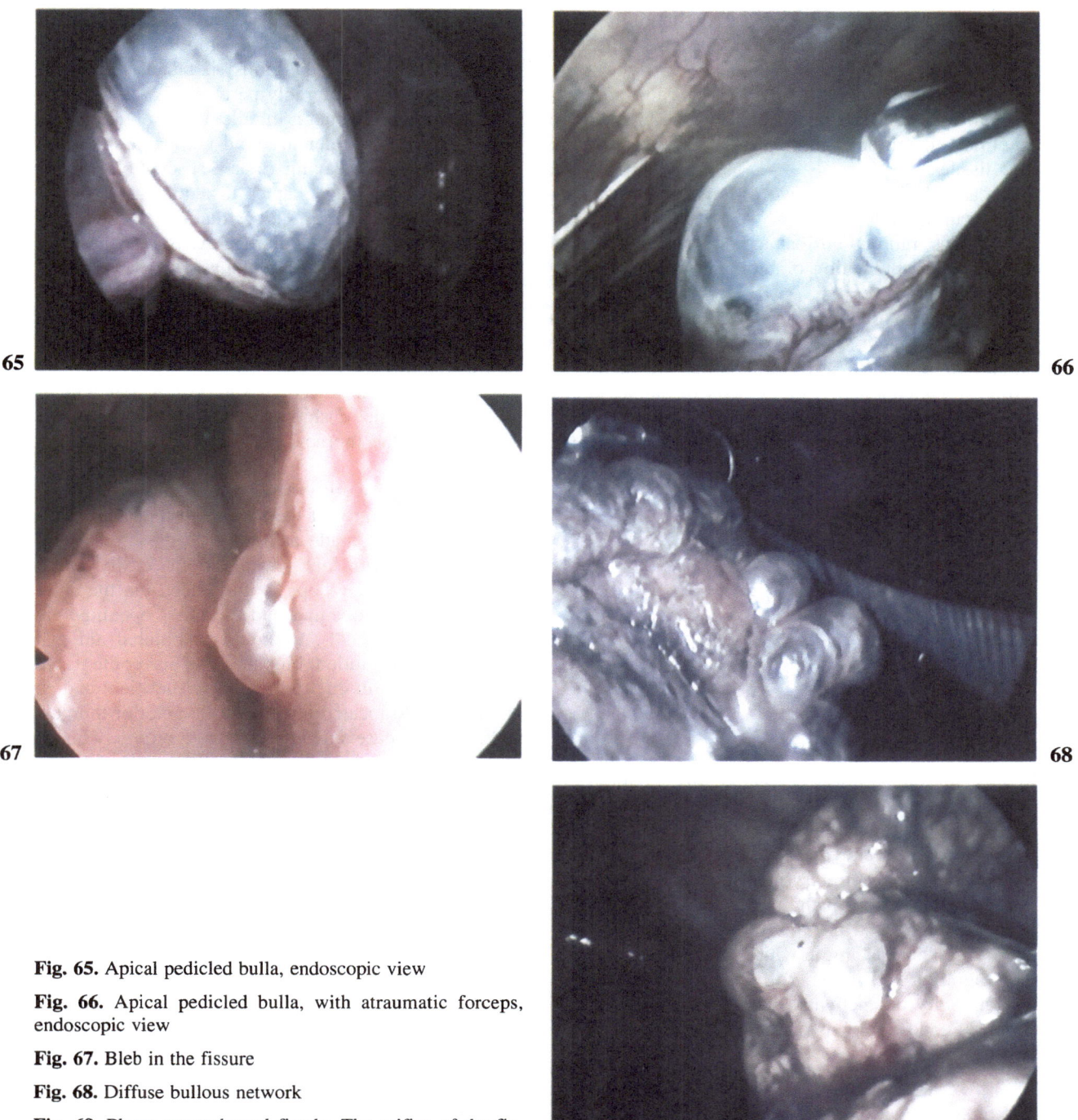

Fig. 65. Apical pedicled bulla, endoscopic view

Fig. 66. Apical pedicled bulla, with atraumatic forceps, endoscopic view

Fig. 67. Bleb in the fissure

Fig. 68. Diffuse bullous network

Fig. 69. Pleuro-parenchymal fistula. The orifice of the fistula can be seen at the top of the bulla

Lung resection is checked by a ventilation test that allows a search to be made for air leaks, the best treatment of these leaks being preventive. Lung resection must be done as much as possible in areas of healthy parenchyma where the staples ensure maximal airtightness in relation to the dystrophic lung tissues.

In case of air leakage, two different circumstances may occur, as follows:

– there is minimal air leakage of alveolar origin: in this case the application of biologic glue to the row of staples is useful;

– there exists major air leakage linked to a tear in the parenchyma or to a poorly stapled distal bronchiole; in this case airtightness must be achieved through application of further rows of staples or by manual suturing using a resorbable thread, this carried out under video control in the thorax via the posterior opening.

3.2. Pulmonary resection and interstitial pathology

One must differentiate between lung biopsy of an excluded lung, where it is easy to choose the site(s) of biopsy according to preoperative information, and biopsy of a ventilated lung in patients with chronic respiratory insufficiency who cannot tolerate selective intubation.

3.2.1. Preliminary aspects

In this special pathologic context, the technique of endoscopic surgery must take into account certain factors, such as the following:

– the pulmonary disease is chronic, with or without chronic respiratory insufficiency;

– the parenchymal pathology is diffuse but heterogeneous (Fig. 76) while the aim of biopsy is to obtain a fragment of lung in which lesions are present;

– the lung is fragile with hepatized, rigid and inflammatory parenchyma, that may tear upon application of endoscopic instruments.

3.2.2. Technical consequences

The type of positioning (i.e. lateral or dorsal decubitus) and the possibility of lung exclusion by selective intubation is governed by the patient's respiratory status. Ideally, the lateral thoracotomy position remains the best since it permits complete examination of the lung as well as easy access to the mediastinum and its lymph nodes.

The localisation of lesions in preoperative CT-scans best determines the site for lung biopsy (Fig. 77). In this pathologic context, the biopsy must be large enough to yield a diagnosis but not result in a significant loss of lung parenchyma. Preoperative intravenous lung scintigraphy indicates the least functional side, where the biopsy is taken.

Lung biopsy is preferably performed at the tip of a lobe (lingula, Nelson or middle lobe) or along the edge of a lobe in order to avoid taking samples that are too thick and leaving tissues susceptible to tearing on application of staples to a thick and fragile hepatized parenchyma. This situation is especially frequent when infectious disease exists. For the same reasons, one must avoid making wedge resections when interstitial disease is present. If the lung is ventilated (i.e. patient with respiratory insufficiency not able to tolerate lung exclusion) then the technique is very different:

– the patient is placed in supine position with if possible a parallel cushion under the thorax, in order to disengage the thoracic wall on the side of operation.

– the surgeon works within a narrower visual field due to the proximity of the ventilated lung parenchyma. Biopsies are made at the tip of the lingula, the middle and inferior lobes, which are all easily accessible areas. The telescope is introduced via the anterior axillary line opening and the other openings are also anterior (Fig. 78). It should be pointed out that thoracic video-guided biopsies in this context are dificult to perform due to the poor visual field and an operative field located just under the anterior thoracic wall. In this case an anterior thoracotomy with or without resection of a costal cartilage, certainly remains an easy and rapid procedure in this particular context.

3.3. Pulmonary resection and tumors

3.3.1. Preliminary aspects

At the present time, endoscopic thoracic surgery is only indicated for diagnosis and treatment of peripheral tumors of the lung (Fig. 79).

In fact, the first-step dissection of thoracic blood vessels is presently feasible, in patients with a free fissure and favorable anatomy. But in the majority of patients, the thoracic vessels (pulmonary veins, branchs of the pulmonary artery or main pulmonary artery) are obscured by lymph nodes.The high risk of vessel injury during vascular dissection, without bleeding control, is currently the main obstacle to safe lobectomy by endoscopic thoracic surgery. As a consequence, endoscopic carcinologic excision is not yet possible.

The indications for endoscopic thoracic surgery are the ablation and diagnosis of a peripheral tumor or the rare cases presenting bilateral lesions that

Fig. 70. CT scan: voluminous bullae

Fig. 71. Endoscopic view of a giant bulla (> 15 cm) with its vascular network

Fig. 72. Opening the bullous lesion using electrocoagulating scissors, note adhesion between bulla and chest wall

Fig. 73. Giant bulla collapsed

Fig. 74. Localisation of the implantation base of a giant bulla

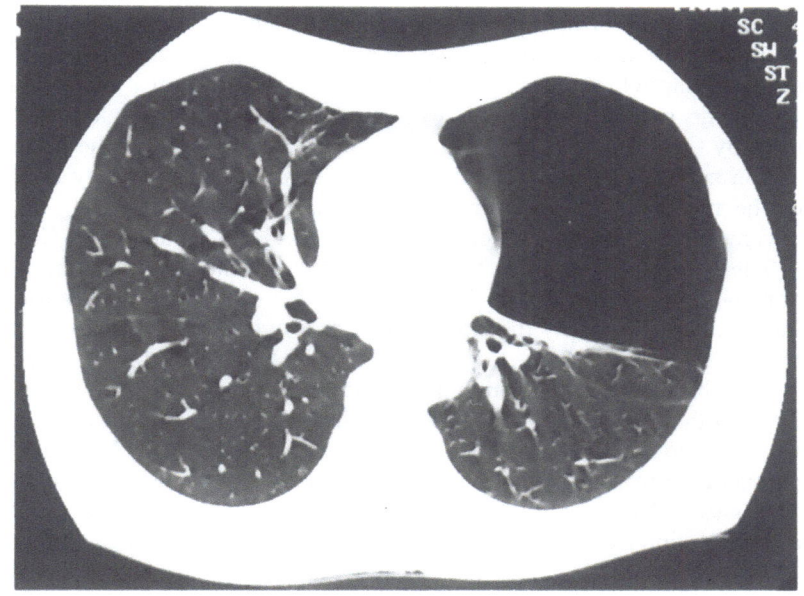

70

71

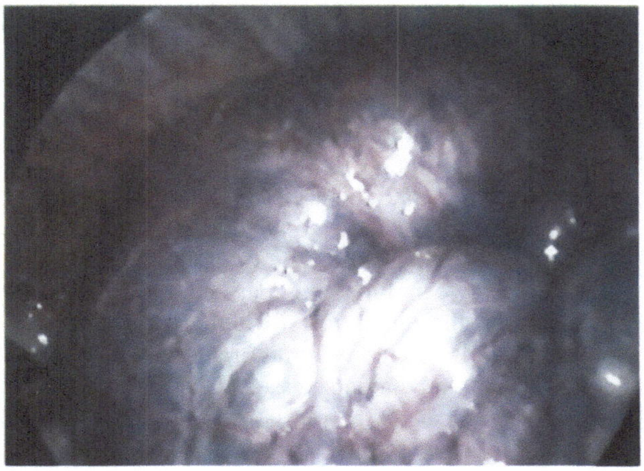

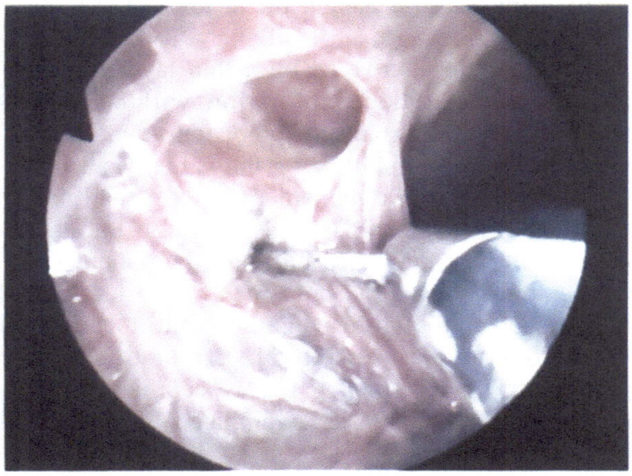

72

73

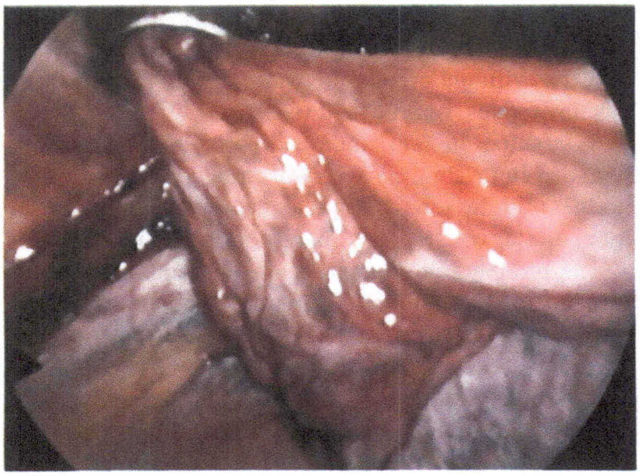

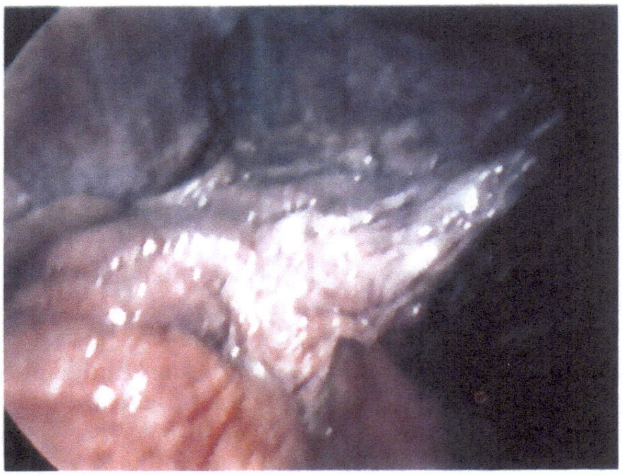

74

create problems in therapeutic management. Surgery of metastases is conceivable but requires complete eradication, which might be difficult to confirm when one considers the underestimation of metastases by CT-scan.

The surgery itself is not difficult, but localisation of the nodule(s) creates a problem, especially when covered by healthy lung parenchyma.

The larger the nodule, the less feasible is the approach with automatic forceps, and the more important it is to apply the stapler away from visible lesions.

The absence of preoperative histologic information requires that excision be made in a healthy area, with a systematic exploration of the mediastinum and with peroperative frozen section available if needed.

In cases of benign solid tumors, one can perform an enucleation by dissection flush with the tumor.

3.3.2. Technical factors

Visual exploration is easy if the lesion is a subpleural one (Fig. 80).

If the nodule is covered by a thin layer of parenchymal tissue, video exploration will be useless (Fig. 81). The importance of preoperative localisation must be stressed, emphasizing the value of all localisation procedures such as anteroposterior and profile chest x-rays, thoracic CT-scans, and also the usefulness of a CT-scan carried out with the patient in the thoracotomy position accompanied by the marking of the skin at points corresponding to the locations of the lesions to be operated [2]. Exploration is then performed via an opening made according to cutaneous reference marks in a ventilated lung which is subsequently excluded.

In some cases, the lesion to be biopsied cannot be found, so it may be useful to enlarge the posterior opening by 3 cms to allow digital palpation.

According to the topography of the nodules to be resected, the entry sites may be modified. Only the posterior opening is always the same, since it permits exploration of the entire thoracic cavity, including all of the lobes and may be enlarged by several centimeters if necessary.

The other two trocars are placed triangularly with respect to the posterior opening (i.e. with an axillary base for lesions of the superior hemithorax) (Fig. 82) and with a diaphragmatic base for lesions of the inferior lobe (Fig. 83) or with an anterior base for anterior inferior nodules (Fig. 84). The distances between the various openings are adapted according to patient corpulence and the length of the endoscopic instruments (the longer they are, the greater the distance between openings).

The type of resection performed depends on the

position of the nodule with respect to the borders of the lobe. If the nodule is close to the tip or the edge of a lobe, a linear resection is adequate. In the other cases a wedge resection will be necessary (Fig. 85).

In the absence of preoperative histologic information, any doubt as to the possible presence of a primary lung tumor calls for immediate histopathologic analysis. Confirmation of this possibility requires thoracotomy so that carcinologic treatment of the primary lung tumor can be performed.

In case of solid benign tumor (e.g. hamartochondroma), an enucleation is performed. After localisation of the lesion, electrocoagulation of the visceral pleura and parenchyma covering the tumor is carried out. Next, the lesion must be stretched out either by using forceps or by traction on a figure-8 thread passed into the lesion. Only progressive dissection in contact with the tumor then remains to be done by electrocoagulation using a coagulating hook or an endoscopic dissector.

Excision of peripheral tuberculoma (Fig. 86) is a good indication for operative thoracoscopy. Clinical experience distinguishes two groups of tuberculomas:

– the apical nodule of quiescent tuberculosis raises the question of the differential diagnosis between tuberculoma and malignant disease.

In this location, endoscopic excision is difficult and frequently impossible. The tight and hemorrhagic adhesions between lung and parietal or mediastinal pleura render the dissection difficult and even hazardous as regards the large intrathoracic vessels (superior vena cava, subclavian vessels) or phrenic nerve. Endoscopic apical dissection is often completed by a short lateral thoracotomy (video-assisted thoracotomy).

– non-apical peripheral tuberculoma involves different problems, presenting as a peripheral lesion with or without preoperative diagnosis. Under these circumstances operative thoracoscopy gives excellents results. In fact, there are often few adhesions between lung and chest-wall in tuberculomas located in the middle lobe or apical segment of the lower lobe, and a wedge resection is possible (Fig. 87).

The preoperative diagnosis of tuberculoma therefore calls for caution. The operative field must permit classical thoracotomy in order to complete a difficult apical dissection. Trocar incisions will be located either at the future incision of a lateral thoracotomy or future drainage openings. Despite these restrictions, endoscopic thoracic surgery presents numerous advantages: it permits avoidance of a thoracotomy for a benign peripheral lesion or may reduce considerably the extent of thoracotomy for apical tuberculoma.

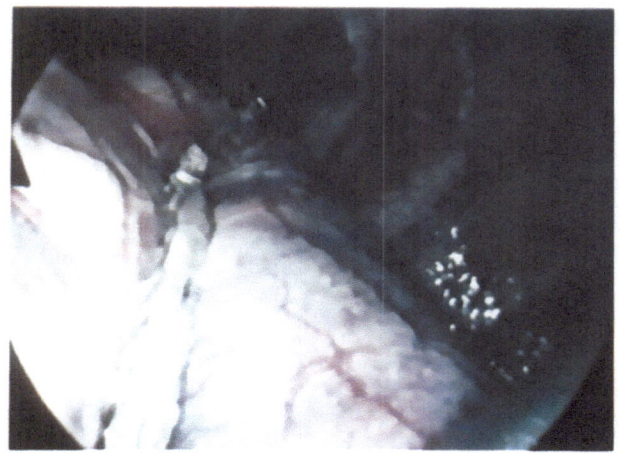

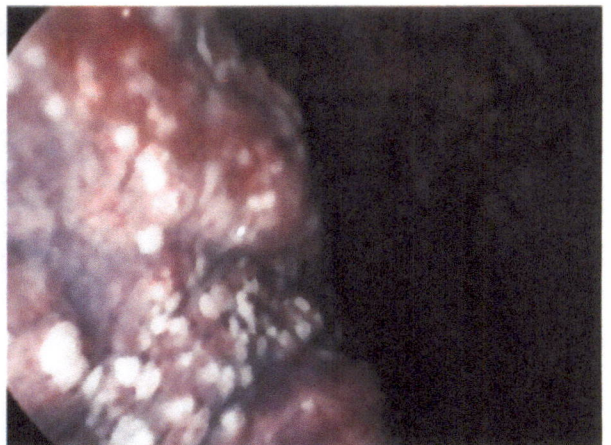

75

76

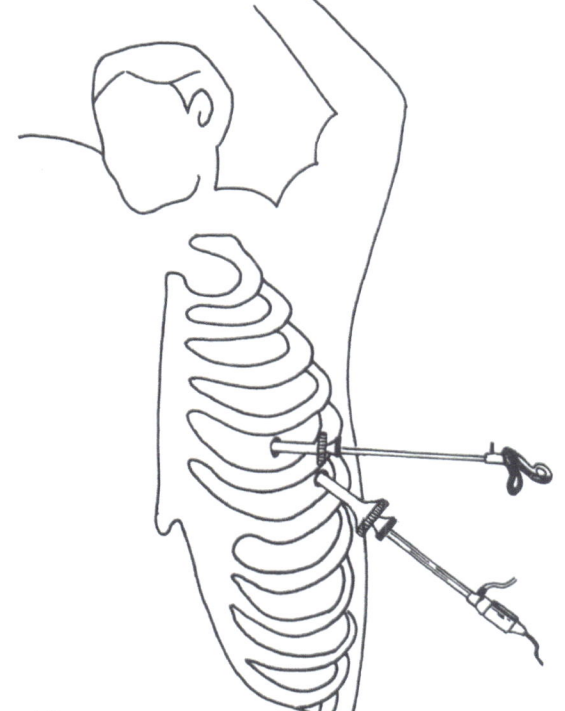

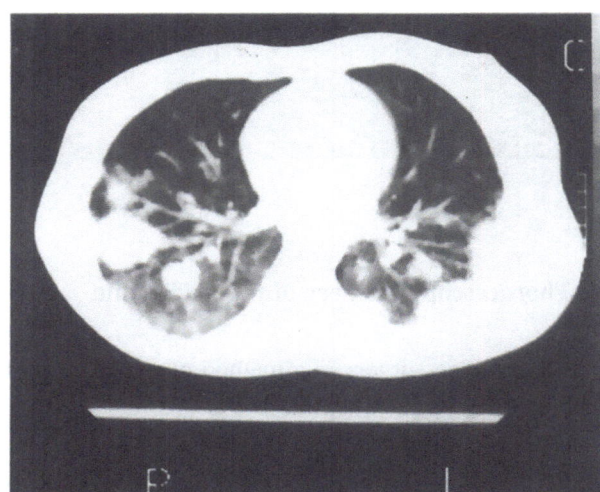

77

78

Fig. 75. Endoscopic view after stapling resection

Fig. 76. Endoscopic view of pneumocystosis in AIDS; diagnosis was made by lung biopsy during endoscopic pleurodesis for bilateral pneumothorax

Fig. 77. CT scan of lung sarcoidosis

Fig. 78. Openings for patient with respiratory insufficiency unable to tolerate lung exclusion or for pericardial exploration

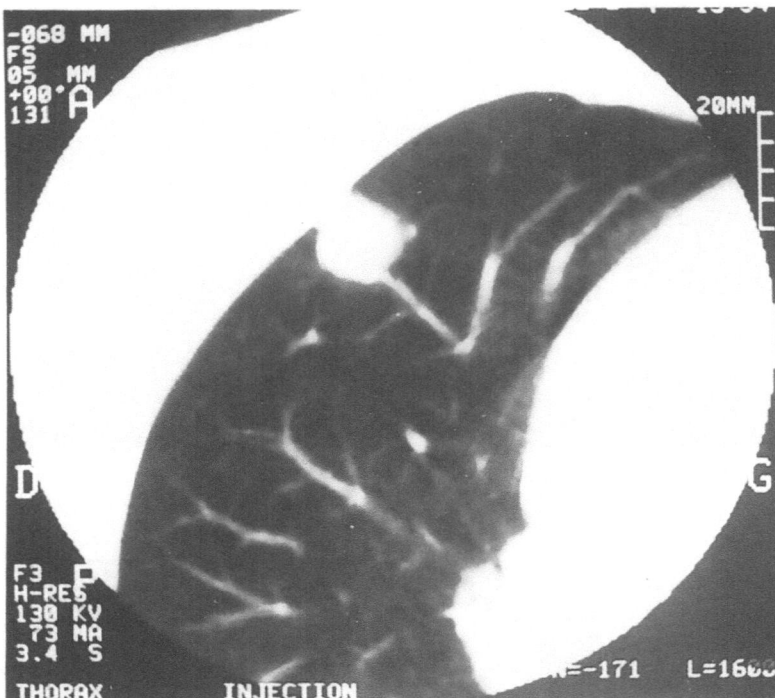

Fig. 79. CT scan of a peripheral tumor treated by endoscopic wedge resection; it was a tuberculoma

4. Thoracoscopic surgery of the mediastinu

Thoracic video-surgery is a method of exploration of the mediastinum whose indications are especially represented by lymphatic lesions.

The paratracheal lymphatic trunks must be explored by mediastinoscopy, which is the method of choice.

Operative thoracoscopy is useful when this method cannot be used due either to a tracheotomy (mediastinoscopy is impossible) or the need to access the posterior mediastinal lymphatics or the inter aortico-pulmonary window (Fig. 88), both of which are characterised by difficult accessibility.

Thoracic video-surgery is also indicated when one wants to combine a lung biopsy with lymph node biopsies. It is also possible in the presence of a superior vena cava syndrome.

4.1. Preliminary aspects

There are two major types of mediastinal lymphatic pathology: either there exist lymphatic metastases of a tumor of the lung, or a primary lymphatic disease (lymphoproliferative lesions), for which no histopathologic information is available. In the latter case, thoracic video-surgery aims to make the diagnosis and define the extent of disease. Operative endoscopy permits excision of tissue specimens of adequate size in order to carry out examinations determining the exact type of lesion.

Secondary lymphadenopathic masses are often voluminous and inflammatory. They present adhesions to the mediastinal surface of the lung.

All of these mediastinal structures are covered by the mediastinal pleura which can be inflammatory, thickened and hemorrhagic, thus masking the subjacent anatomic elements. This is especially found in cases of lymphadenopathic metastases of a primary tumor of the lung. The major risk of this surgery is an injury to a mediastinal vascular structure such as the superior vena cava, the arch of the azygos vein, the pulmonary artery or even the aortic arch. The anatomic relationships here may be disturbed in the presence of a voluminous tumoral mass. For lesions of the posterior mediastinum the risk is an injury to the esophagus.

These risks therefore call for the application of certain basic guidelines, which are outlined in the following paragraphs.

One must have a good preoperative idea of the anatomic relationships between the lesions to be operated and the vascular elements of the mediastinum; this is obtained through thoracic CT-scan with injection.

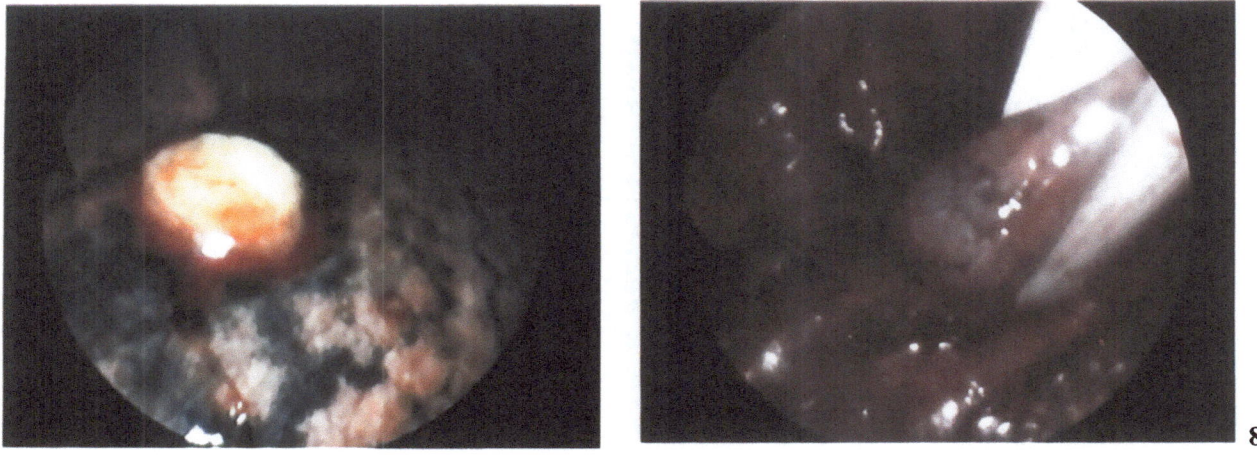

Fig. 80. Peripheral lung nodule

Fig. 81. Subpleural nodule covered by a thin layer of parenchymal tissue, in the jaws of the Endo Gauge

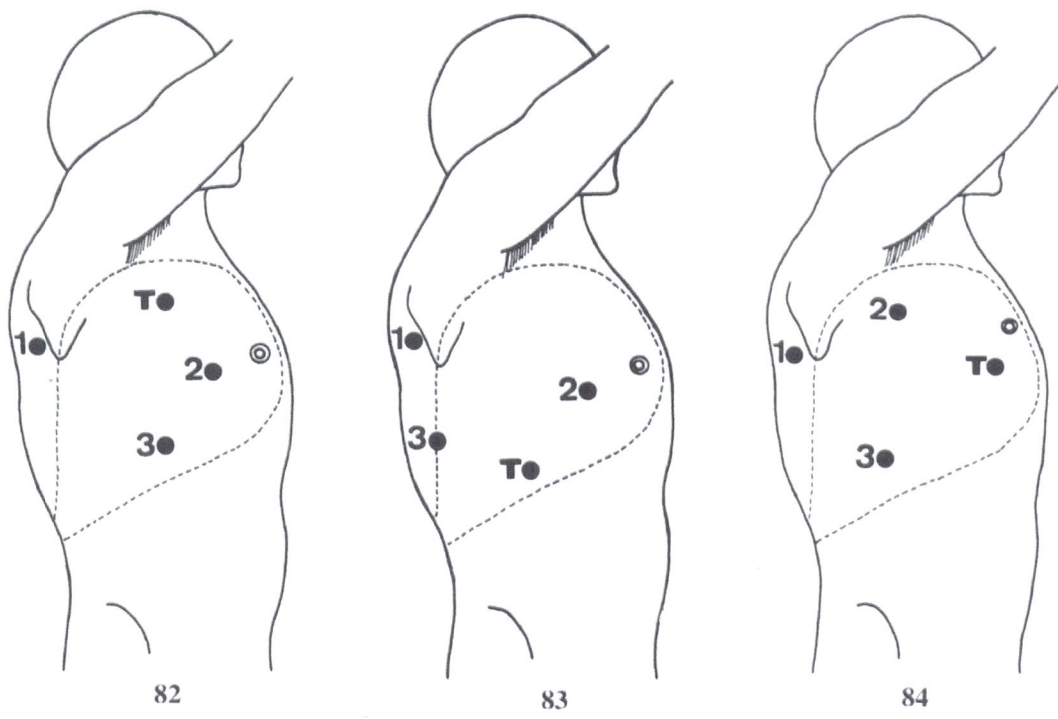

Fig. 82. Three openings forming a triangle with an axillary base for an apical tumor (T)

Fig. 83. Three openings forming a triangle with an inferior base for a basal tumor (T)

Fig. 84. Three openings forming a triangle with an anterior base for an anterior tumor (T)

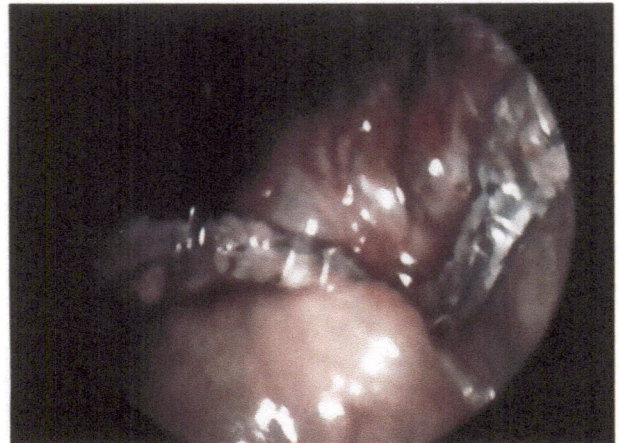

Fig. 85. Wedge resection

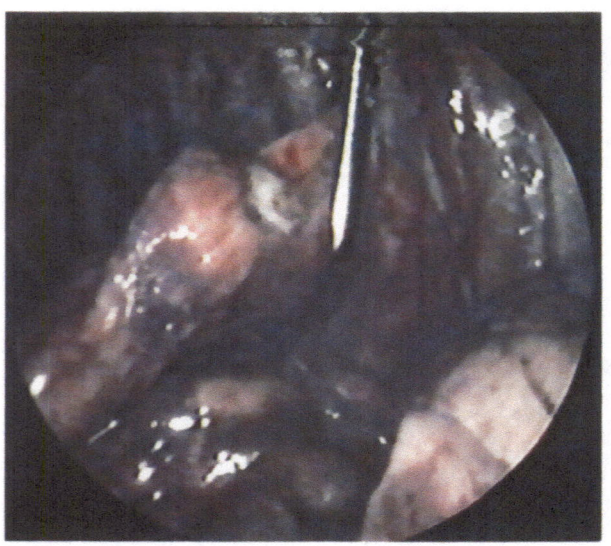

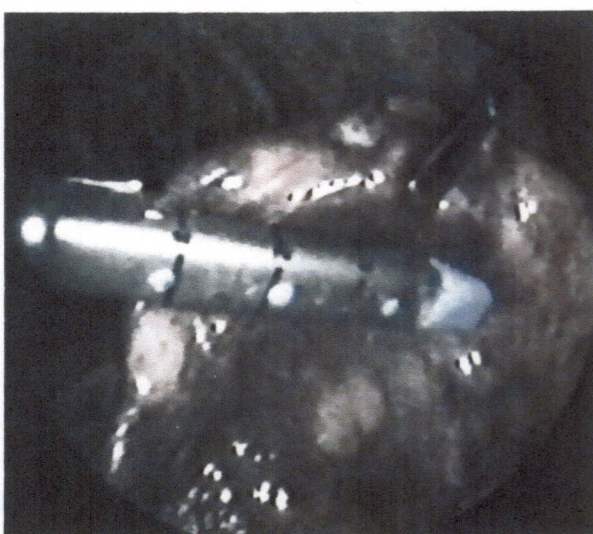

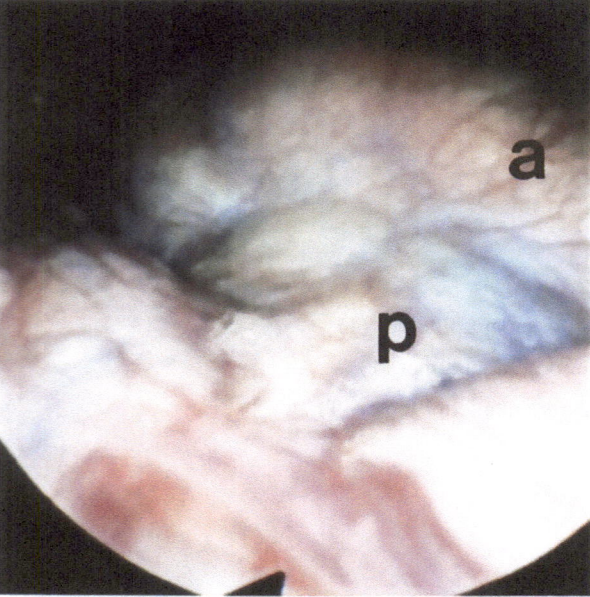

Fig. 86. Peripheral tuberculoma located on the edge of the middle lobe

Fig. 87. Wedge resection of a peripheral tuberculoma (Fig. 86)

Fig. 88. Endoscopic view of the aortico-pulmonary window. *a* aortic arch. *p* left pulmonary artery

The careful lysis of pleuroparenchymal adhesions is an essential step leading to a large operative field with a good exposure of the mediastinum.

It is always necessary to open the mediastinal pleura before performing biopsies. Repetitive irrigation is valuable in very inflammatory hemorrhagic lesions for better visualisation. When the lesion is contiguous with a vascular structure as evidenced by CT-scan, dissection at a distance from the area of contact and aspiration before any biopsy is necessary.

4.2. Technical factors

Installation in the lateral thoracotomy position is required. The operation is always performed using three openings that form a triangle. It is often necessary for exploration of the superior mediastinum (Fig. 89) to situate one of the ports in the axillary region in order to avoid operating in a tangential fashion on the lesions. A supplementary opening for placement of a lung retractor may prove very useful.

In case of primary lymphadenopathic pathology, an excision of a lymph node is possible by dissection in contact with the lymph node. On the other hand, in other cases only extensive biopsies are taken.

Thoracic video-surgery also permits confirmation and removal of certain benign mediastinal tumors and thus avoids an unnecessary thoracotomy.

Cystic disorders such as paraesophageal or bronchial cysts (Fig. 90) are ideal indications for thoracic video-surgery. These lesions are always easily removed from the thorax through one of the trocar tubes after their puncture. They are benign, thus not requiring lymphatic dissection which is difficult to perform under thoracoscopy. The real problem is that of discerning indications, especially for pleuropericardial cysts or mediastinal lipomas (Fig. 91). The positioning of the patient and the entry sites do not present any particular problem. The approach is often an easy one since there are no or few adhesions between the mediastinum and the lung. The cyst must be totally removed. Exposure may be improved by aspiration of the cyst. Dissection must be done in contact with the lesion in order to avoid injuring adjacent structures such as the phrenic nerve when a pleuropericardial cyst is present, or the vagus nerve when a para-esophageal cyst exists, or the œsophagus and subcarinal lymph nodes with bronchial cysts (Fig. 92). Exposure may be facilitated in some cases by dividing the azygos vein using a vascular endostapler. A cystic collar may be left when adhesions exist between a bronchial cyst and the tracheobronchial membrane. No specific problems are noteworthy concerning the surgery of paraesophageal or paratracheal cysts.

Surgical thoracoscopy permits the bacteriologic diagnosis and evacuation of paravertebral tuberculous spindle-shaped sequestrations. This is indicated only in the absence of diagnosis by the usual procedures or if there is a threat of cutaneous fistulization despite the correct management of medical treatment. The operation is a simple one to perform. The patient is placed in the lateral position. After exposure of the posterior mediastinum, the laterovertebral cradle pouch is opened (often after previous aspiration with a large caliber trocar) and the sequestration is removed using a curette. Two drains are installed for postoperative irrigation and washing.

5. Thoracoscopic surgery of the pericardium

Surgical thoracoscopy may be useful in certain cases of pericardial effusion. In this chapter concerning technique, we will not discuss indications but only the procedure of pericardotomy. Two situations are possible, as follows:

– a symptomatic neoplastic pericarditis with tamponade (Fig. 93).

In this context, the patient must remain in the semi-reclining position and the drainage treatment begins under local anesthesia. In the absence of associated pleural effusion, or if the pericardial effusion is slight in quantity, the opening for entry will be made into the left pleural cavity. If not, we use the side with associated pleurisy (which will have been previously drained). After local anesthesia, the first trocar is introduced on the anterior or mid-axillary line according to the size of the cardiac silhouette at the level of the 4th or 5th intercostal space (Fig. 78). Routine examination of the pleural cavity is made. Next, the pericardium is reached by pushing aside the lung or through the left fissure (Fig. 94). A minute opening in the pericardium is made with scissors introduced via the optic operative channel in order to relieve the tamponade. A second trocar is introduced into the subjacent intercostal space for use of forceps. A pericardial window (Fig. 97) is then made in order to avoid a short-term recurrence. The phrenic nerve is always localized in order not to injure it during the pericardotomy (Figs. 95, 96). If a neoplastic pleurisy exists a talcage of the pleural cavity may be associated. A drain through one of the openings is placed and left there for several days.

– a chronic pericarditis of undetermined etiology.

Thoracoscopy permits exploration and biopsy of the pericardium (Fig. 97). This is, however, only feasible when a pericardial effusion is present, even if it is minimal. Chronic constrictive pericarditis is a

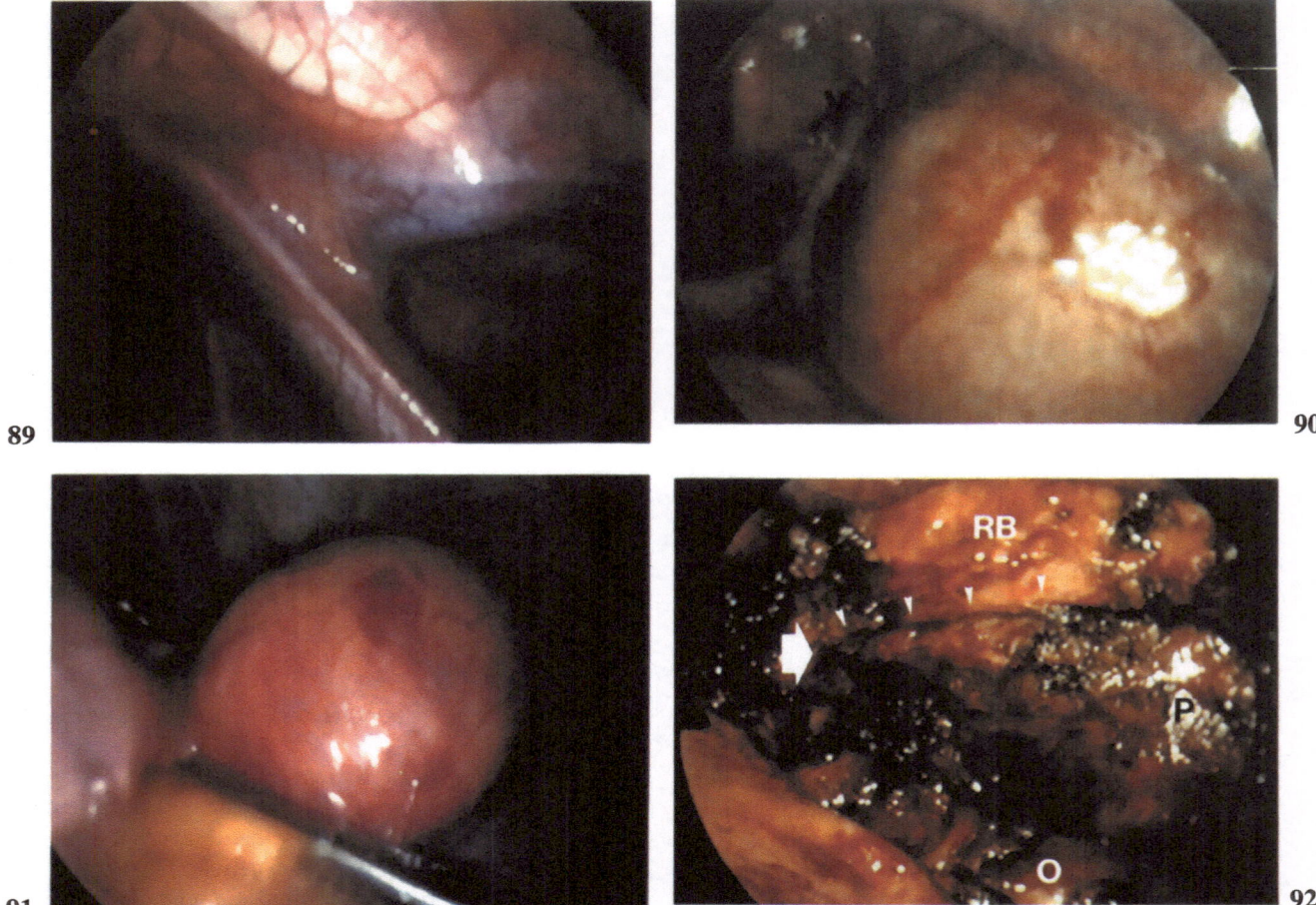

Fig. 89. Endoscopic view of the right upper mediastinum; superior vena cava, right phrenic nerve

Fig. 90. Endoscopic view of a bronchial cyst stretching the azygos vein *(V)*

Fig. 91. Cardio-phrenic lipoma

Fig. 92. Endoscopic view of subcarinal area after complete excision of a bronchial cyst. *White arrow :* carina, *small arrows* : inferior edge of the right bronchus *(RB), P :* pericardium, *O :* œsophagus

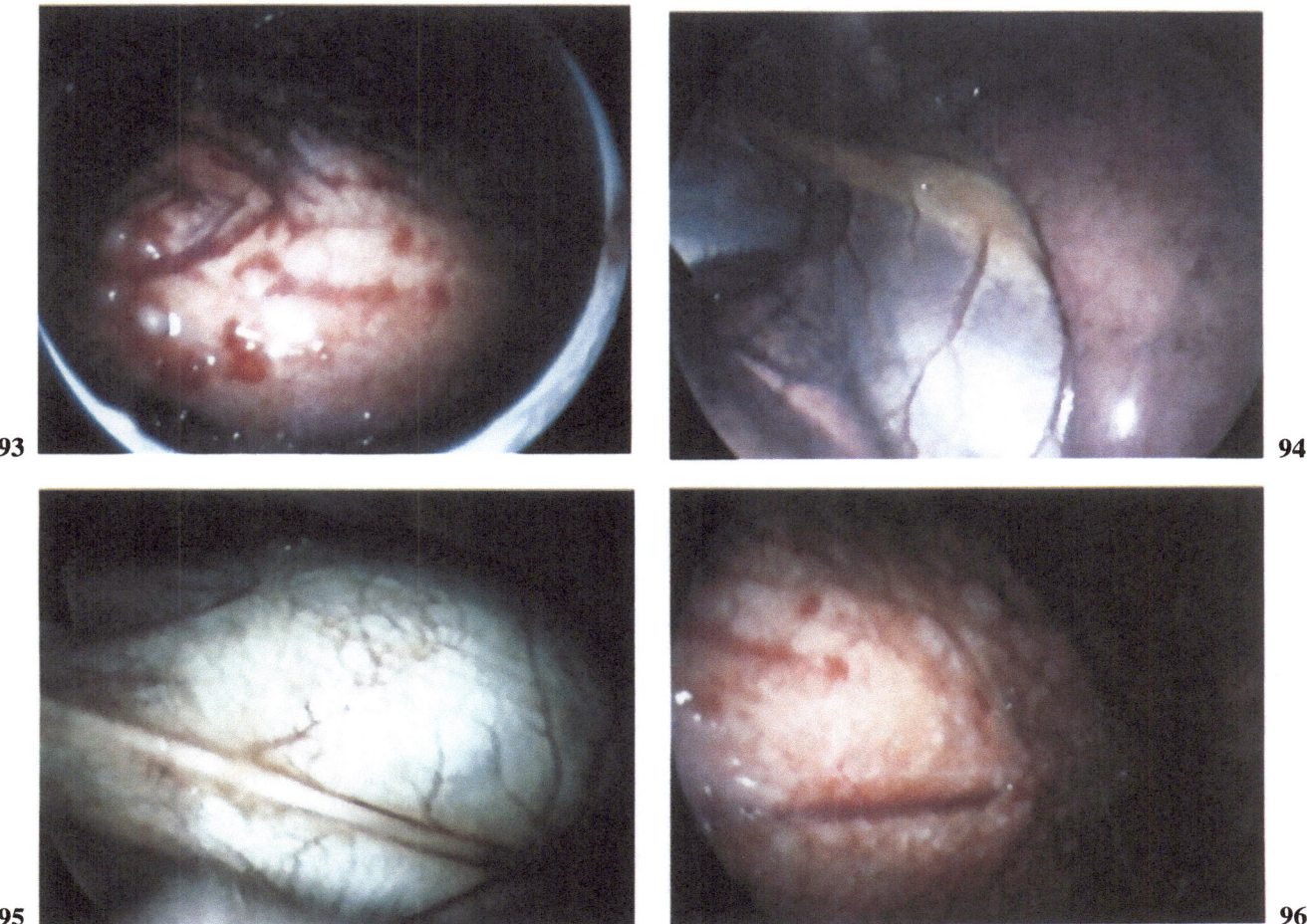

93

94

95

96

Fig. 93. Neoplastic pericarditis with tamponnade

Fig. 94. Pericardium is reached through the left pulmonary fissure

Fig. 95. Localisation of the phrenic nerve on healthy pericardium

Fig. 96. Localisation of the phrenic nerve on neoplastic pericardium

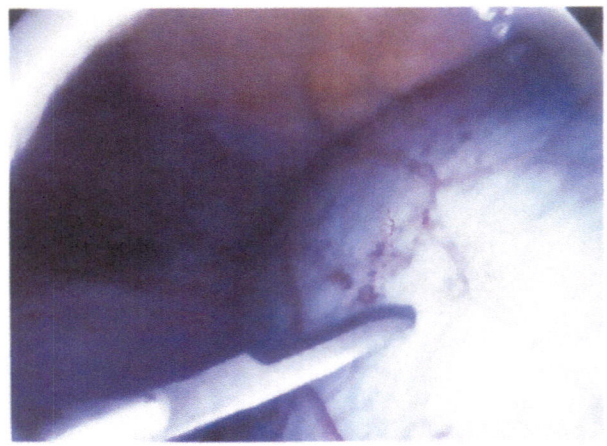

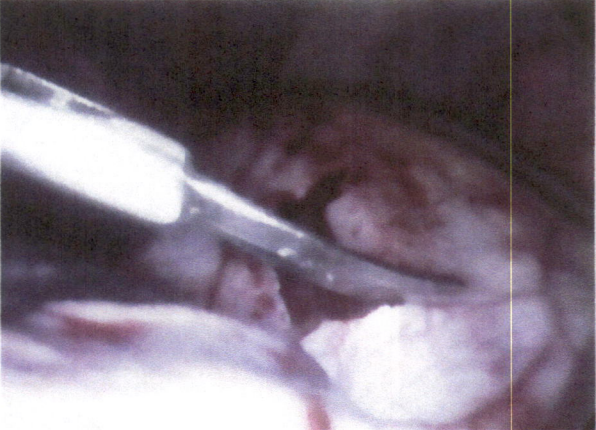

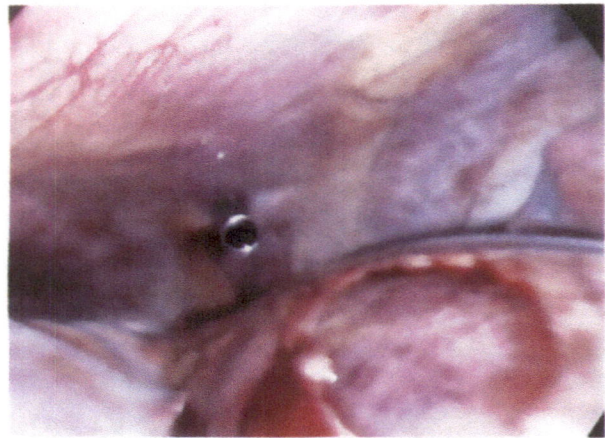

Fig. 97a-c. Pericardial window for pericarditis. **a** Puncture of the pericardium using endoscopic micro-knife. **b** The window is made using endoscopic scissors. **c** View of the pericardial window below the phrenic nerve (Photographs : D. Gossot)

contradication to these percutaneous techniques, due to the adhesions between the pericardium and underlying myocardium. The operation is carried out under general anesthesia with the patient either sitting or in the thoracotomy position.

6. Chest wall and miscellaneous aspects

Sometimes the preoperative diagnosis of chest wall tumor is obvious as in tumors of the posterior mediastinum (costovertebral cradle) (Fig. 98).

In some cases, with parietal contact of the tumor evidenced in the CT-scan, the diagnosis is only suggested and thoracic video-surgery leads to differen-

tiation of a parietal tumor from a peripheral lung tumor.

In surgery of parietal tumors (Fig. 99), it is essential to individualise and diagnose neurinomas preoperatively. Any extension into the intervertebral foramen (neurinoma forming an intraspinal protuberance) requires preliminary neurosurgery. This intravertebral extension must be searched for routinely through x-ray films focused on the inter-vertebral foramina, a thoracic CT-scan and especially by MRI. An artery of Adamkiewicz whose origin is just outside an intervertebral foramen must be searched for in an arteriogram, especially if the neurinoma is a lower one.

Preparation of the patient is as usual. The openings are located according to the lesions topography. An axillary opening is useful in order to avoid operating

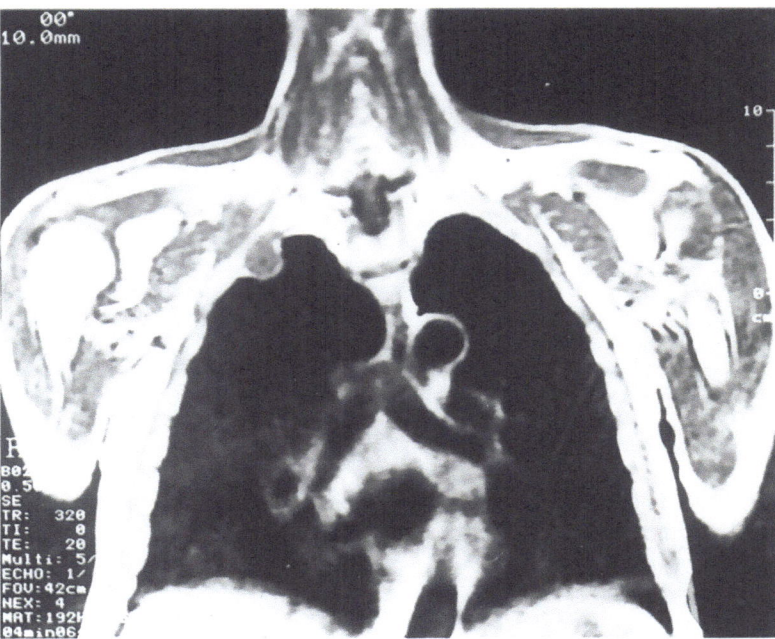

Fig. 98. MRI of an apical neurogenic tumor

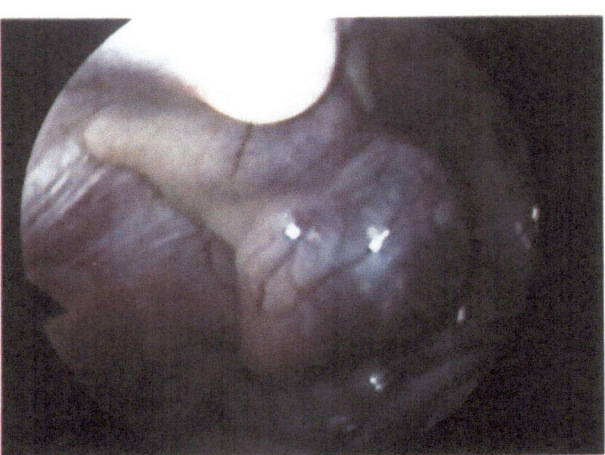

Fig. 99. Chest wall schwannoma

tangentially when superior lesions are present. In neurogenic tumors, dissection must stay in contact with the lesion to protect adjacent structures (Fig. 100), with localisation of the upper and lower nerve trunks which are clipped, then sectioned (Fig. 101). It may be expedient to leave the parietal pleura covering the tumor in place in order to facilitate its mobilisation and dissection. For other lesions, (such as fibroma) the resection is made at a distance from the primary lesion in healthy tissue.

7. Conclusion

Strides in technology have promoted endoscopic thoracic surgery procedures. Initially reserved for pleural surgery, thoracic video-surgery now extends its field of application to thoracic pathology. Diagnosis and excision of peripheral lesions of the lung and of some mediastinal or parietal tumors, and performance of lung biopsies or biopsies of voluminous lym-

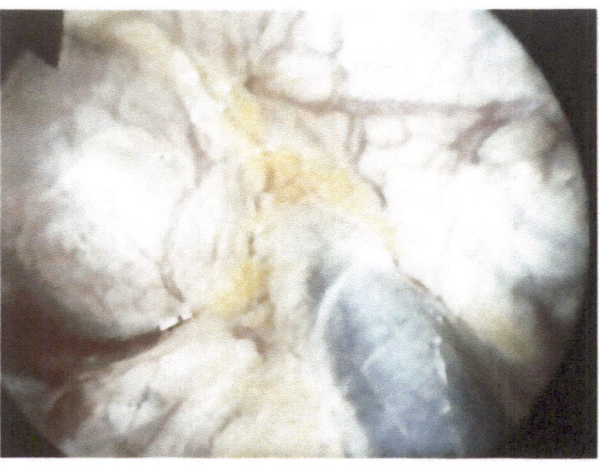
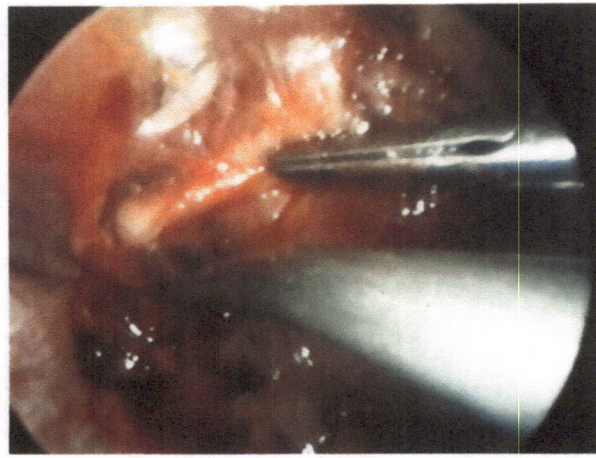

100   101

Fig. 100. Apical neurinoma closely adherent to the superior vena cava

Fig. 101. Nerve trunk of a chest-wall neurinoma

phadenopathic nodules, are the most prominent reasons supporting the role that endoscopic thoracic surgery plays today. As it permits surgery without resorting to thoracotomy, endoscopic thoracic surgery should become one of the techniques available to the thoracic surgeon.

References

1. Boutin C, Viallat JR, Cargnino P, Rey F (1982) Thoracoscopic lung biopsy. Chest 82 : 44-48
2. Daly B et al (1991) Computed Tomography-Guided Minithoracotomy for Resection of Small Peripheral Pulmonary Nodules. Ann Thorac Surg 51 : 465-469
3. Dijkman JH, Van der Meer JWM, Bakker W et al (1982) Transpleural lung biopsy by the thoracoscopic route in patient with diffuse interstitial pulmonary disease. Chest 82 : 76-83
4. Kleinmann P, Levi JF, Debesse B (1991) La pleurectomie parietale percutanée par vidéo endoscopie. Le traitement moderne du pneumothorax spontané récidivant. Rev Mal Resp 8 : 459-462
5. Levi JF, Kleinmann P, Riquet M, Debesse B (1990) Percutaneous parietal pleurectomy for recurrent spontaneous pneumothorax. Lancet 336 : 1577-1578
6. Nathanson LK, Shimi S, Wood R, Cuschieri A (1991) Videothoracoscopic ligation of bulla and pleurectomy for spontaneous pneumothorax. Ann Thorac Surg 52 : 316-319
7. Wakabayashi A (1989) Thoracoscopic ablation of blebs in the treatment of recurrent or persistent pneumothorax. Ann Thorac Surg 48 : 651-653
8. Wakabayashi A et al (1991) Thoracoscopic carbon dioxide laser treatment of bullous emphysema. Lancet 337 : 881-883

Thoracoscopic treatment of empyema thoracis

P.D. Ridley

1. General considerations

Empyema thoracis is of historical interest to the thoracic surgeon as it represents the first intrathoracic pathology to be treated surgically [7]. Improved antibiotic treatment has resulted in a reduction in the incidence of empyema thoracis [5] and an alteration in the responsible pathogens [1, 11, 19]. However empyema thoracis remains a condition with a significant morbidity and mortality [10]. Although antibiotics are effective in treating pneumonia and have therefore reduced the incidence of empyema, their value in established non-tuberculous empyema with frank pus in the pleural cavity is unproven [11]. Early, adequate drainage with subsequent sterilization of the pleural cavity remains the essential principle in successful management. Re-expansion of the lung reduces the size of the empyema space, improves chances of resolution and is desirable, but not essential. It is rarely possible to close a postpneumonectomy empyema space but it can be sterilized. Empyema is usually recognized and treated initially by the chest physicians using multiple aspirations or closed [underwater seal] drainage. In some cases, such conservative management results in successful resolution. However, this often proves inadequate and patients who are referred to thoracic surgeons usually represent failures in medical management. It is advisable for all cases of empyema to be treated surgically at an early stage [19]. Surgical approaches include rib resection and open drainage [11, 15], open window thoracostomy [2, 3], decortication [8], thoracoplasty [6, 18], intrathoracic muscle transposition [13] and cyclical irrigation [16].

Thoracoscopy with [15] or without [4, 21] cyclical irrigation of the thoracic cavity has also been descri-bed in the management of empyema thoracis. Postpneumonectomy empyema has also been managed thoracoscopically [12]. However, few units employ this technique routinely and its role remains controversial.

Thoracoscopy is usually performed under general anaesthesia with the patient in the lateral position. A double lumen tube allows the lung on the affected size to collapse, improving visualization of the empyema cavity. Inflating the cuff around the endo-bronchial tube to the good lung is important to avoid spillage from the empyema cavity in the event of a bronchopleural fistula. Of course, patients who have undergone previous pneumonectomy are intubated with a standart single lumen tube cut long to allow the inflatable cuff to be placed below the carina. It is useful to insert a Saugmann's needle (GU instruments, London, England) into the empyema cavity to determine its extent and locate a dependent site where the lung is displaced from the chest wall and unlikely to be damaged by instrumentation. Typically the fifth intercostal space in the posterior axillary line is chosen. It has been our practice to employ a standard laparoscope/thoracoscope. The large bore of this instrument allows better debridement. Its superior lighting and field of view and its offset parallel eyepiece allows easier manipulation of the biopsy forceps and suckers.

2. Assessment of lung expansibility

Empyema classically begins as an infection of a low viscosity pleural effusion with an underlying lung which is fully expansile. Subsequently the fluid becomes more turbid and a thin layer of fibrin starts

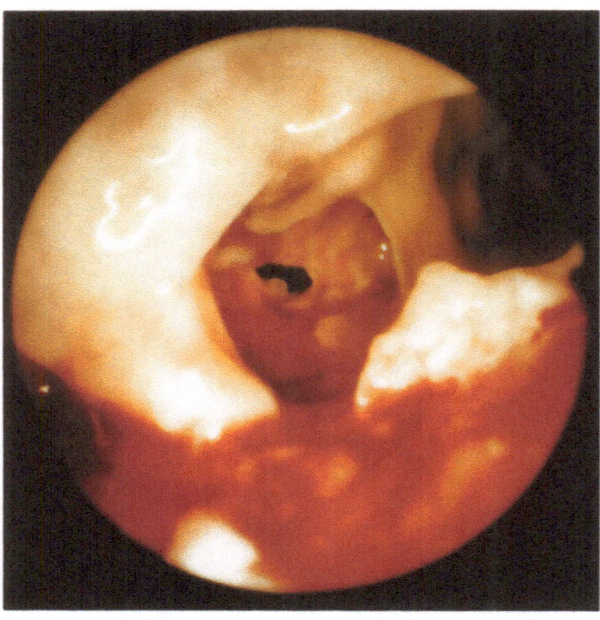

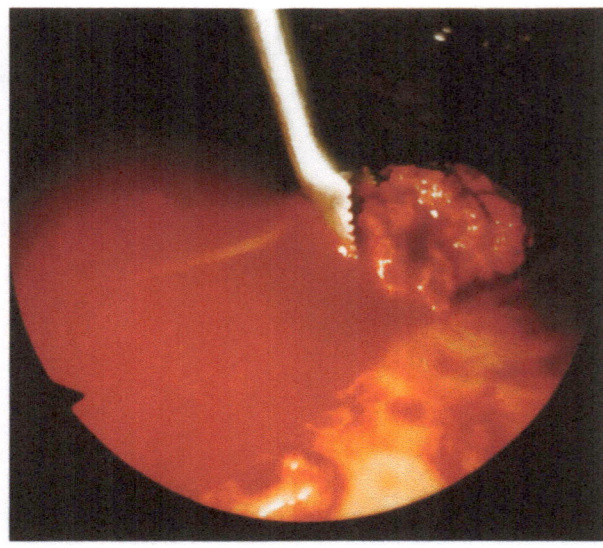

Fig. 102. Thoracoscopic view of an empyema thoracis (Photograph : D. Gossot)

Fig. 103. Thoracoscopic removal of necrotic tissues, using an endoscopic scraper (Photograph : D. Gossot)

to cover the lung and pleural surface. Further organization occurs as fibroblasts and capillaries invade the fibrin peel covering the lung and pleural surfaces. Eventually, a thick fibrous walled cavity containing viscous pus is produced and expansion of the underlying lung is extremely limited (Fig. 102). This process typically takes place over a period of six weeks. The transition from a thin-walled fibrin-covered cavity containing thin infected pleural effusion to a thick, fibrous-walled cavity containing viscous pus represents a spectrum of pathological conditions. The patient may be seen at any stage of the condition. The expansibility of the underlying lung may be assessed at thoracoscopy. Thus some indication of further management requirements may be obtained. These findings may alter treatment, distinguishing patients with early empyema likely to resolve with thoracoscopic debridement and tube drainage [15, 20] from those with late empyema and a non-expansile lung which might benefit from decortication.

3. Debridement

Thoracoscopy allows full debridement [and thus adequate drainage] because with the tip of the instru-

ment and long-handled forceps loculi of pus and adhesions can be broken down under direct vision (Fig. 103). The empyema cavity can be repeatedly washed out with warm saline during the procedure. Full debridement is possible because of the wide bore of the thoracoscope canula, with any debris that becomes lodged in the canula being readily removed with long-handled forceps.

4. Drain placement and post-operative irrigation

Accurate drain placement, impossible to determine by roentgenography alone, is ensured by drains being positioned under direct vision. Thus, dependent drainage can be ensured. If postoperative pleural irrigation [15] is employed an apical 12 F Argyle drain can be placed under direct vision for infusion of irrigation fluid. The thoracoscope is replaced with a 32 F basal Argyle drain wich fits the hole made by the thoracoscope trocar without drainage leaking around it. Sideholes cut in the basal drain allow drainage over a 15 cm length of tube, with the lowest hole 2,5 cm inside the parietal pleura. The advantages of the Argyle drain is that at 37°C it is supple and is tolerated intercostally for weeks if necessary. If open drainage subsequently becomes necessary, this can sometimes be achieved by simply shortening the basal drain without rib resection.

The technique of repeated irrigation ensures that the basal drain is effectively dependent. Thoracoscopy combined with cyclical irrigation should not be considered a success only if complete resolution is obtained by this technique alone. Rapid symptomatic improvement is obtained by removal of pus and infected material such that the patient is better able to withstand subsequent surgical interventions. This is particularly obvious when a bronchopleural fistula is present.

A bronchopleural fistula would make complete resolution with thoracoscopic debridement and pleural irrigation very unlikely and it becomes apparent when the patient notices the salty taste of the irrigation fluid. Smaller volumes of irrigation fluid and alteration of the patients position is required to continue irrigation. However, the patient is rapidly rendered less toxic and better able to withstand subsequent surgical intervention. In our department in a series of 30 patients, complete resolution was obtained by this technique alone in 18/30 (60 %). Of the 12 patients in whom complete resolution was not obtained, 5 had bronchopleural fistulas. Secondary surgical measures resulted in resolution of empyema in 8. Four patients died; all were elderly, severely debilitated, and 3 had advanced malignancy [15].

5. Biopsy

Thoracoscopic biopsy has been shown to be an effective method for diagnosing malignancy which reduces the need for formal diagnostic thoracotomy [9]. The aetiology of empyema is frequently in doubt, particularly in patients who are debilitated and unable to give a clear history. Thoracoscopy allows routine multiple pleural biopsies under direct vision in all patients with empyema. Thus, the chances of overlooking an underlying malignancy, such as mesothelioma, are minimized.

6. Foreign bodies

As well as malignancy thoracoscopy may reveal previously unsuspected underlying aetiologies for empyema. In an early description of the merits of thoracoscopy in the management of empyema, Weissberg [21] described a patient in whom thoracoscopy revealed a surgical sponge which had been left in the pleural cavity during a coronary artery bypass operation 2 years earlier. It was possible to remove the foreign body with the thoracoscope resulting in complete resolution of the empyema. In a second patient, Weissberg describes thoracoscopic identification of pus and undigested food particles in the right pleural cavity and made the diagnosis of a previously unrecognized perforation of a malignant tumor of the esophagus. Segments of retained polyethylene catheters may be identified radiologically and removed thoracoscopically [12].

7. Conclusion

Thoracoscopy is a relatively atraumatic procedure which, with modern anaesthesia, is well tolerated in severely debilitated patients. It allows easy determination of lung expansibility and a search for factors underlying the empyema. Thorough debridement with removal of pus results in rapid resolution of the patient's toxicity and accurate, dependent drainage is possible under direct vision. Subsequent surgical procedures are not precluded by this atraumatic technique and it is hoped that the relatively non-invasive nature of the surgery involved will encourage physicians to refer cases of empyema thoracis directly to a thoracic surgeon. Early thoracoscopy should be considered in patients presenting with empyema thoracis.

References

1. Barlett JG, Gorgach SL, Thadepalli H, Finegold SM (1974) Bacteriology of empyema. Lancet 1 : 338-340
2. Bayes AJ, Wilson JAS, Chiu RC, Errett LE, Hedderich G, Munro DD (1987) Clagett open-window thoracostomy in patients with empyema who had and had not undergone pneumonectomy. Can J Surg 30 : 329-331
3. Cicer R, Del Velccho C, Porter JK, Carreno J (1986) Open window thoracostomy and plastic surgery with muscle flaps in the treatment of empyema thoracis. Chest 89 : 374-377
4. Cronen PW, Alcorn GL (1985) Use of thoracoscopy in the management of empyema thoracis. Indiana Med 78 : 1012-1013
5. Elving G (1954) A comparison of the frequency of lung abcess, pneumonia, acute bronchitis and acute pleural empyema. Acta Chir Scand 107 : 454-455
6. Gregoire R, Deslauriers J, Beaulieu M, Piaux M (1987) Thoracoplasty: its forgotten role in the management of nontuberculous postpneumonectomy empyema. Can J Surg 30 : 343-345.
7. Hippocrates (1965) In Major classic description of disease. Edited by C. Thomas. Springfield, IL
8. Hoover EL, Hsu HK, Ross MJ, Gross AM, Webb H, Ketosugbo A, Finch P (1986) Reappraisal of empyema

thoracis surgical intervention when the duration of illness is unknown. Chest 90 : 511-515

9. Hucker J, Bhatnagar NK, Al-Jilaihawi AN, Forrester-Wood CP (1991) Thoracoscopy in the diagnosis and management of recurrent pleural effusions. Ann Thorac Surg 52 : 1145-1147

10. Lemmer JH, Botham MJ, Orringer MB (1985) Modern management of adult thoracic empyema. J Thorac Cardiovasc Surg 90 : 849-855

11. Neild JE, Eykyn SJ, Phillips I (1985) Lung abscess and empyema. Quart J Med 57 : 875-882

12. Oakes DD, Scherck JP, Brodsky JB, Mark JBD (1984) Therapeutic thoracoscopy. J Thorac Cardiovasc Surg 87 : 269-273

13. Pairolero PC, Arnold PG, Trastek VF, Meland NB, Kay PP (1990) Postpneumonectomy empyema: the role of intrathoracic muscle transposition. J Thorac Cardiovasc Surg 99 : 958-968

14. Ridley PD, Braimbridge MV (1991) Thoracoscopic debridement and pleural irrigation in the management of empyema thoracis. Ann Thorac Surg 51 : 461-464

15. Ridley PD, Myers C, Braimbridge MV (1989) Empyema thoracis. Professional Nurse (Vov) 73-76

16. Rosenfeldt FL, McGibney D, Braimbridge MV, Watson DA (1981) Comparison between irrigation and conventional treatment for empyema and pneumonectomy space infection. Thorax 36 : 272-277

17. Sang CTM, Braimbridge MV (1981) Thoracoscopy simplified using the laparoscope. Thorac Cardiovasc Surg 29 : 129-130

18. Sarkar SK, Sharma TM, Singh A, Purohit SD, Sharma VK (1985). Thoracoplasty with intercostal myoplasty for closure of an empyema cavity and bronchopleural fistula. Int Surg 70 : 219-221

19. Smith JA, Mullerworth MH, Westlake GW, Tatoulis J (1991) Empyema thoracis: 14-year experience in a teaching centre. Ann Thorac Surg 51 : 34-38

20. Wakabayashi A (1991) Expanded application of diagnostic and therapeutic thoracoscopy. J Thorac Cardiovasc Surg 102 : 721-723

21. Weissberg D (1981) Pleuroscopy in empyema: is it ever necessary? Poumon-Cœur 37 : 269-272

Thoracoscopic sympathectomy

J. Byrne, T.N. Walsh and W.P. Hederman

1. Introduction

Of all the procedures performed by the operative tho-
racoscopist, few can match the success or wide
acceptance of endoscopic sympathectomy. As a minimally invasive surgical technique, it incorporates
improved cosmetic, ready patient acceptability, and
shorter hospital stay with demonstrably fewer complications than "open" procedures. Indeed, the evolution of surgical thoracic sympathectomy mirrors that
of minimally invasive surgery over the past 30 years.
Such are the advantages of endoscopic sympathectomy, that the time has surely arrived when familiarity
with the technique should be a prerequisite for all
surgeons routinely performing upper thoracic sympathectomy.

Today, the major indication for surgical sympathectomy remains the treatment of palmar and axillary hyperhidrosis refractory to medical management.
Causalgia, the term referring to burning pain often
accompanied by increased sweating following trauma
to an extremity, can also be successfully treated by
adequate surgical sympathectomy [1], although chemical sympathectomy remains the more usual
method of treatment. Its role in the management of
previously accepted conditions such as Raynaud's
disease and peripheral vascular disease of the upper
limb is surely no longer tenable in light of its poor
overall results in these settings [2, 3], while indications such as epilepsy [4], spastic paralysis [5] and
arthritis [6] are interesting only as historical foot-
notes. Four operative approaches to sympathectomy
remain in common usage, each with its advocates: 1)
the cervical or supraclavicular approach, 2) the transaxillary or transthoracic approach, 3) the dorsal or
posterior midline approach, and 4) transthoracic electrocautery (TTEC) or perhaps more accurately, endoscopic or thoracoscopic sympathectomy.

2. Historical perspective

Since the first description of successful excision of
part of the sympathetic chain in an epileptic patient
by Alexander in 1889, the procedure of surgical sympathectomy and its indications have evolved considerably. Jaboulay in 1899 was the first to describe the
vasomotor implications of successful surgical sympathectomy. However the first description of cervical
sympathectomy for vascular disease was by Janesco
and Brunning in 1923. In 1928, Royle described the
operation of sympathetic "reamisection" for Raynaud's disease and spastic paralysis of the upper
limb by an inverted T incision [7]. Gask in 1933 described the commonly used transverse incision [8]
whilst Adson in 1935 described a single stage cervical approach in the management of hyperhidrosis [9].
Adson and Brown, in 1929, described a posterior
approach involving removal of portions of two ribs
on either side allowing exposure of the sympathetic
chain [10], although even by the standards of the
1930s, this was regarded as being a somewhat traumatic alternative to the less invasive anterior approach [6]. Cloward, however, revived interest in this
approach in 1969 with his description of a dorsal
approach using a single incision, allowing access to
both sides and involving partial resection of one or
two ribs on either side [11]. Indeed this technique or
modifications of it involving bilateral costotransversectomy of the third rib still remain in vogue amongst
neurosurgeons in North America and several have
reported quite large series using this approach with

good results [12, 13]. Atkins in 1949 was the first to report his experience with a peraxillary transpleural approach [14], although it has the disadvantage of always requiring two separate operations and mandatory insertion of a chest drain. In addition, cosmetic results have not always been ideal with up to 29% of patients expressing dissatisfaction in one series [15].

The first significant report of a standardised technique for thoracoscopic sympathectomy was by Kux in 1954 [16], who reported his results for 1,400 procedures, although inadequacy of instruments and light sources in earlier years must have been a significant problem. Initially, the procedure was performed as a two stage procedure under light sedation without anesthesia and involved surgical excision of the sympathetic chain and its removal with a grasping forceps. This was later modified by Hederman who performed the operation under general anesthesia using a double lumen endotracheal tube [17], which allowed each lung to be selectively deflated and re-inflated in a sequential manner and permitted completion of both sides at the same sitting. An additional modification was the substitution of unipolar diathermy for the grasping forceps and cauterisation of the chain. A further refinement to allow both diathermy and operating laparoscope to be introduced through the same incision was abandoned due to postoperative rib pain.

3. Indications and patient selection

The main indication for operative sympathectomy, regardless of the approach, is primary or "essential" palmar and axillary hyperhidrosis. Hyperhidrosis is a pathologic condition in which sweating occurs in excess of that required for normal thermoregulation. The total daily loss in these patients may reach up to 12 liters in extreme cases. Epidemiologic data in the English literature are scant, but Adar suggests an incidence in Israel of 0.6-1.0% [18]. Hyperhidrosis may be primary, with no obvious cause, or secondary to a variety of neurologic or systemic diseases such as thyrotoxicosis, pheochromocytoma and diabetes mellitus. Symptoms most often appear at puberty, but may date back to early childhood and persist throughout adult life. It is usually localised to the palms, axillae and feet, but the face, back, groin, and legs may also be affected. Not surprisingly, hyperhidrosis can severely interfere with the patient's lifestyle, markedly restricting both social and professional activities and is especially inconvenient for those whose work entails dealing with the public. Indeed, perhaps the best known, albeit inadvertent, characterisation of a hyperhidrotic subject was by Dickens in

his description in *David Copperfield* of Uriah Heep: " ... his damp cold hand felt so like a frog in mine that I was tempted to drop it and run away... He took out his pocket-handkerchief, and began wiping the palms of his hands" [19].

Hyperhidrosis, in common with a great many other medical conditions is not an "all or nothing" phenomenon but spans a spectrum from those with quite mild degrees of palmar and axillary sweating who can be managed adequately by conservative measures to those with severe degrees of sweating and for whom surgery offers the only hope of relief. In a review of our experience in the Mater Misericordiae Hospital, Dublin of 112 patients operated for this condition only a third of all patients were of sufficient severity to warrant operative treatment [20]. The remaining two thirds either responded to non-surgical measures such as topical application of 15 or 20% aluminium chloride hexahydrate antiperspirant solutions or had a significant psychological component.

The role of operative sympathectomy in the management of Raynaud's disease has fallen into disrepute in the last decade and although anecdotal reports exist of its benefit in individual cases, long term follow-up of these patients has proven disappointing [20]. Relapse following successful sympathectomy may occur at any time and is believed to be due to the high local reactivity of blood-vessels in and the early return of autonomous vascular tone [21]. The patient is frequently left with the added disappointment of uncomfortably dry hands as a result of sudomotor denervation. We have now largely abandoned this procedure for severely affected patients in the past in favor of more conservative measures.

4. Technique

4.1. Preoperative investigations

Preoperative preparation and investigation are essential for all patients undergoing thoracoscopic sympathectomy. Routine laboratory and radiologic screening tests, including full blood count, erythrocyte sedimentation rate (ESR), urea and electrolyte estimation, blood-glucose, thyroid function studies and chest radiography, are carried out to preclude an underlying cause. As this is essentially an elective procedure for a non-life threatening condition, albeit a quite distressing one, it is essential that patients be carefully counselled on potential complications of the operation such as postoperative pain, possible pneumothorax requiring insertion of a chest drain and the very real possibility of some degree of compensatory

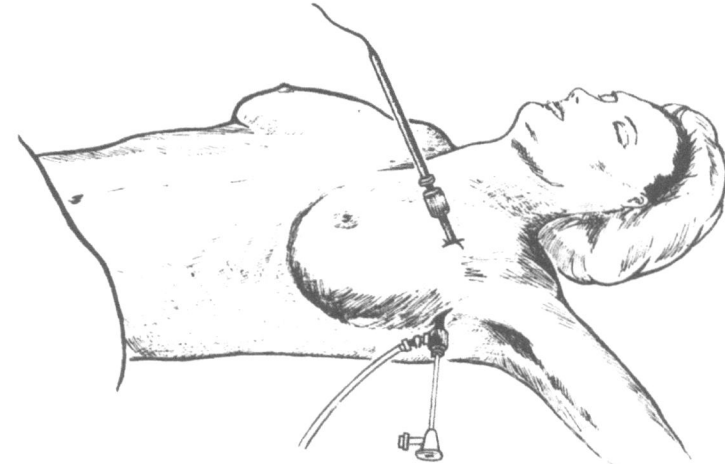

Fig. 104. The position of the patient on the operating table demonstrating the sites of insertion of the operating thoracoscope and unipolar diathermy

hyperhidrosis in other areas of the body, previously unaffected. Patients with a clinical history suggesting pleural adhesions or radiologic evidence of pleural thickening are not offered this procedure, although this is not usually a problem in these rather young patients.

4.2. Surgical technique (Fig. 104)

The procedure is performed under general anesthesia using a double lumen endotracheal tube. The patient is placed in the supine position with both arms abducted to 90°. Blood-pressure and heart-rate are monitored throughout the operation. An artificial pneumothorax is established by insufflating 0.5 litres of CO_2 through a Verres needle in the 4th intercostal space, having first disconnected the ipsilateral portion of the endotracheal tube from the ventilator. A small incision is made in the 4th intercostal space in the anterior axillary line and a laparoscope is introduced through a cannula. More CO_2 is introduced and the upper lobe of the lung is observed as it collapses. Flimsy adhesions will often be encountered at this stage and can be safely cut with a diathermy scissors. Major apical adhesions may be difficult to cut and quite vascular and may even render the operation impossible.

The sympathetic chain is usually visualised under the parietal pleura running down over the necks of the second to sixth ribs (Fig. 105). A unipolar diathermy probe is inserted through a separate stab incision, usually in the midclavicular line. If the chain is not easily seen due to subpleural fat it can be located by stroking the diathermy along the neck of the rib. The chain is then felt and seen as it slips out from under the tip of the probe. The pleura over the chain can be incised with diathermy and the second, third, and fourth thoracic ganglia and intervening chain are now electrocoagulated until they present a charred appearance. This differs from the technique of Kux and others [16] who, at this stage of the operation, attempted to remove the chain with a grasping forceps and dissecting scissors. If axillary hyperhidrosis is also a problem, then it is advisable to also remove the fifth ganglion for adequate denervation of the axilla. Stellate ganglion injury is not a problem when using the thoracoscopic technique as it is covered by a characteristic yellow fat pad and not visualised at operation.

On completion of the first side, the endotracheal tube is reconnected and the lung is reinflated, allowing CO_2 to escape through the cannula. Reinflation of the lung is then checked through the laparoscope and when fully inflated, the procedure is repeated on the opposite side under the same anesthetic. This has caused no problems in our experience, many surgeons still prefer to perform it as a two stage procedure, especially where close postoperative monitoring may be a problem. It is important that pulse rate and blood pressure be monitored carefully throughout the entire operation to guard against inadvertent pneumothorax, and the CO_2 line pressure should not exceed 10 cm H_2O. The whole procedure from start to finish in experienced hands takes no longer than 30-35 min.

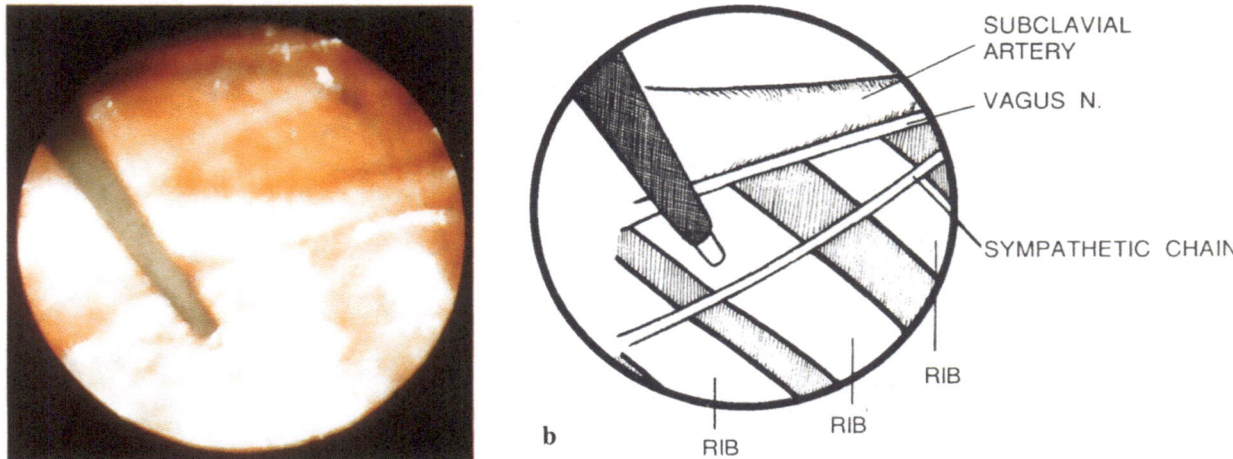

Fig. 105a, b. The sympathetic chain as seen **a** through a thoracoscope and **b** as a line diagram

A chest radiograph is performed on all patients in the recovery room after the operation and must always be viewed prior return back to the ward. Chest drains are not routinely placed unless there is a specific indication such as troublesome oozing that cannot be contained by direct pressure or a significant pneumothorax. These occur only rarely in our experience. A further chest radiograph is performed 24 hours after surgery and the patient is usually discharged on the second postoperative day.

5. Results

Few operations can compare with the dramatic and immediate effects of surgical sympathectomy for palmar and axillary hyperhidrosis. Usually, the success or otherwise of the procedure is quite apparent by the first postoperative day. The main concern of the operating surgeon, however, must be whether or not this is a lasting effect. Certainly the early results suggest that endoscopic sympathectomy provides effective and long term relief with minimal side-effects.

In our own series [20], we reviewed 112 patients, circularising them with a detailed questionnaire, inquiring into all aspects of their condition and how they fared following surgery. In all but one patient, the hands and axillae were recorded as dry on returning from theatre. In one early case the procedure was unsuccessful and had to be repeated. Seventy eight of the 85 patients on whom follow-up was complete reported immediate satisfaction with the procedure (Table 1). There was no mortality and no serious morbidity in our series. Horner's syndrome occurred in three patients, resolving in two within six weeks and in one by six months. Why this should resolve lies in the cause, which we believe to be edema secondary to the inflammatory reaction generated by the process of electrocoagulation. Surgical emphysema was noted in three patients and a pneumothorax requiring a chest drain occurred in one patient. One patient had a wound infection in one of her stab incisions. Other transient postoperative phenomena included chest pains (8 patients), back pains (4 patients), and somewhat paradoxically a transient Raynaud's phenomenon (4 patients). The mean duration of hospital stay was 3.1 days (range 1-7 days).

Long-term results have been equally gratifying. Our mean follow-up period was 43 months (range 3-95 months). Subjective patient assessment of the effectiveness of surgery was impressive (Table 1). Follow-up was greater than 3 years in 47 patients. Only seven patients of all those surveyed reported deterioration in their overall condition when compared to their initial postoperative result and in four of these the symptoms were still better than that at their initial presentation. A further four patients, on the other hand, recorded an improvement over the same period. Patient satisfaction with cosmesis was particularly gratifying with 68 (80%) grading it as 'good', 13 (15%) as 'moderate' and 4 (5%) as 'fair". No patient expressed dissatisfaction with the cosmetic result. Some compensatory hyperhidrosis occurred in 54 (64%) of patients. This persisted in 44 patients, fading in only ten, with a mean fade-out interval of 10.1 months (range 1-30 months). It was less distres-

Table 1. Subjective assessment of the results of thoracoscopic sympathectomy by 85 patients immediately after operation and at a mean follow-up of 43 months (range 3-95 months)

Assessment	Immediately After operation	At follow-up
Very much improved	67	65
Moderately improved	11	7
Slightly improved	3	7
Unchanged	2	2
Worse	2	3

sing than the original sweating in the majority of patients but it did warrant further investigation and treatment in four patients which accounted for the reported worsening of their overall condition. Of note is that 12/54 patients had some degree of gustatory sweating.

These results are very much in keeping with those of other authors using this technique. Kux [16] reported his experience using their two-stage technique in the treatment of 63 patients and reported no incidence of either pneumothorax requiring a chest drain, surgical emphysema, Horner's syndrome, or wound infection. Of the 59 patients subsequently interviewed, 55 expressed themselves satisfied with the result. In keeping with our own findings, 28 of 63 (48%) of Kux's group of patients reported compensatory hyperhidrosis to some degree, mainly on the trunk, abdomen, and thighs, but this was usually much less distressing than the original condition and in only two patients was this particularly troublesome. Only two patients complained of gustatory sweating.

This experience with endoscopic sympathectomy has been repeated in several other centers. Claes and Gothberg [23] report very similar results in their series, using a slight modification of the technique described above, involving introduction of the Verres needle through a 1 cm stab incision 1 cm under the clavicle and 2 cm lateral to the sternum followed by insertion of a urological resectoscope through the intercostal space. They report that of the 100 cases in their series all were dry after the operation and that at follow-up, 80% reported 'good' results with a further 15% 'improved' and nobody regretting having had the operation. Two patients required insertion of a chest drain, but no other complications occurred.

Banerjee et al [22], in a preliminary communication, seem to have had a similarly satisfactory experience, finding a 95% improvement if only the hands were affected and 77% if both hands and axillae were affected. Thirty eight of their 50 patients descri-

bed some degree of compensatory hyperhidrosis, with 24 mentioning gustatory sweating. Only one of their patients developed a Horner's syndrome which again was only transient.

6. Why thoracoscopic sympathectomy ?

The efficacy of such well established techniques as the cervical, transaxillary, and dorsal approaches to surgical sympathectomy in providing relief from the distressing symptoms of hyperhidrosis cannot be questioned. So why should the surgeon now adopt this newer and more unfamiliar technique? Cervical sympathectomy is probably the most widely practised approach to surgical sympathectomy in Europe but, while undoubtedly effective, it has several not insubstantial drawbacks when compared with the thoracoscopic approach. On a purely technical level, the cervical approach is probably a much more difficult procedure to master, whilst economically the logic of two separate operations involving two hospital admissions when compared with a single 2-3 day stay seems flawed. There is a greater risk of Horner's syndrome, which is a more frequent finding and more likely to be permanent when the cervical approach is utilised. Reported incidence of permanent Horner's syndrome following this procedure varies in the literature from 1% in Keaveny's group [24] to 8% in Adar's series of 100 patients [18], although Adar did report at least a mild degree of Horner's syndrome in 57% of their patients. In addition, brachial plexus contusion has been reported in up to 11% of patients by this approach while up to 6% will have a significant pneumothorax requiring insertion of a chest drain. Although numerous of well documented series are to be found in the literature, very few have specifically looked at satisfaction with cosmesis amongst their patient group, other than to offer broad generalisations such as "no patient expressed dissatisfaction with their result". Cosmesis, however, must be considered an important aspect in the treatment of this condition as we are electively treating a predominantly young and female population for a non-life-threatening disease. The cosmetic result obtained is inevitably better when the thoracocscope is used producing virtually invisible scars.

Cosmesis and the necessity for two operations must also be considered disadvantages of the transaxillary approach to operative sympathectomy. Indeed Sternberg [15], in his 1981 series reported that up to 29% of patients expressed dissatisfaction with their results in terms of cosmesis when this technique was used. As regards cost, it usually requires a longer hospital stay (3-4 days) and two separate hospital admissions. There is also the necessity for insertion of a chest drain.

The dorsal approach widely used in the United States seems to offer real advantages when compared to cervical or transaxillary approaches. As originally described by Cloward [11], it involves a single posterior midline incision with resection of the second and/or third rib on either side. More recent modifications have tended to be somewhat less traumatic and involve a bilateral costotransversectomy of the third rib. In Pillay's series [12], 94% of patients expressed long term satisfaction in terms of improved sweat responses. The mean hospital stay was similar to that for the endoscopic approach, as was the incidence of significant pneumothorax requiring insertion of a chest drain at 1%. As with the thoracoscopic approach, no patient suffered a permanent Horner's syndrome. These are quite excellent results and obviously this is an effective alternative to the endoscopic approach in those patients deemed unsuitable for thoracoscopy. However, endoscopic sympathectomy provides a superior cosmetic result, and obviates the necessity for either rib resection or costotransversectomy while preserving the integrity of the stellate ganglion.

We consider thoracoscopic sympathectomy the treatment of choice for patients requiring operative sympathectomy. The entire procedure takes only 30-35 min to perform, is a skill easily acquired and presents minimal complications in terms of either Horner's syndrome, significant pneumothorax, or brachial plexus contusion. In addition, it is readily acceptable to the patient and most importantly, given that the vast majority of these patients are young, it is very acceptable from a cosmetic point of view. Familiarity with the thoracoscope should be a prerequisite for all those involved in the surgical treatment of palmar and axillary hyperhidrosis.

References

1. Man B, Kraus L, Motovic A (1976) Axillary sympathectomy for upper extremities. Vasc Surg 10 (3) : 138-143
2. Johnston ENM, Symmerly R, Birnistingl M (1965) Prognosis in Raynaud's phenomenon after sympathectomy. Br Med J 1 : 962-964
3. Hall KV, Hillestad LK (1960) Raynaud's phenomenon treated with sympathectomy: a follow - up study of 28 patients. Angiology 11 : 186-189
4. Khanna SK, Sahariah S, Mittal VK (1976) Supraclavicular approach for upper dorsal sympathectomy. Vasc Surg 9 (3) : 151-159
5. Royle ND (1924) The treatment of spastic paralysis by sympathetic ramisection. Surg Gyn Obst 34 : 701-704
6. Ross JP (1933) Sympathectomy as an experiment in human physiology (Hunterian lecture). Br J Surg 21 : 5-19
7. Royle ND (1928) Sympathetic trunk section; a new operation for Raynaud's disease and Spastic paralysis of the upper limb. Med J Austr 2 : 436-439
8. Gask GE (1933) The surgery of the sympathetic nervous system. Br J Surg 21 : 113-116
9. Adson AW, Craig WM, Brown GE (1935) Essential hyperhidrosis cured by sympathetic ganglionectomy and trunk resection. Arch Surg 31 : 794-798
10 Adson AW, Brown GE (1929) Raynaud's disease of the upper extremity: Successful treatment by resection of sympathetic cervicothoracic and 2nd thoracic ganglia and intervening trunk. JAMA 92 : 444-447
11. Cloward RB (1969) Hyperhidrosis. J Neurosurg 30 : 545-551
12. Pillay PK, Awad IA, Little JR, Dohn DF, Bay JW (1989) Upper thoracic sympathectomy for essential palmar hyperhidrosis: Cleveland Clinic experience with 440 cases. Proceedings of the 39th Annual Meeting of the Congress of Neurological Surgeons, p 217
13. Shih C, Wang Y (1978) Thoracic sympathectomy for palmar hyperhidrosis: a report of 457 cases. Surg Neurol 10 : 291-296
14. Atkins HJB (1949) Per axillary approach to the stellate and upper thoracic sympathetic ganglia. Lancet 2 : 1152-1154
15. Sternberg MO, Bakkman S, Kott J, Reiss R (1982) Transaxillary thoracic sympathectomy for primary hyperhidrosis of the upper limbs. World J Surg 6 : 458-463
16. Kux E (1954) Thorakoskopische Eingriffe am Nervensystem. George Thieme Verlag, Stuttgart
17. Horgan K, O'Flanagan S, Duignan JP, Hederman WP (1984) Bicentennial Proceedings of the Royal College of Surgeons in Ireland, pp 1086-1088
18. Adar R, Kurchin A, Zweig A, Mozes M (1977) Palmar hyperhidrosis and its surgical treatment. Ann Surg 186 : 34-41
19. Dickens C (1850) David Copperfield. Penguin Classics, London
20. Byrne J, Walsh TN, Hederman WP (1990) Endoscopic transthoracic electrocautery of the sympathetic chain for palmar and axillary hyperhidrosis. Br J Surg 77 : 1046-1049
21. Dowd PM (1986) The treatment of Raynaud's phenomenon. Br J Dermatol 114 : 527-533
22. Banerjee AK, Edmondson R, Rennie JA (1990) Endoscopic transthoracic electrocautery of the sympathetic chain for palmar and axillary hyperhidrosis (letter). Br J Surg 77 : 1435
23. Claes G, Gothberg C (1991) Endoscopic transthoracic electrocautery of the sympathetic chain for palmar and axillary hyperhidrosis (letter). Br J Surg 78 : 760
24. Conlon KC, Keaveny TV (1987) Upper dorsal sympathectomy for palmar hyperhidrosis 74 : 651

Thoracoscopic surgery of the esophagus

D. Gossot

Until now, endoscopic dissection of the esophagus has mainly been performed laparoscopically [11, 23]. However, extensive dissection of the esophagus is also feasible through the thoracoscope [16]. In this field, contrary to lung surgery, almost all of the techniques usually performed via thoracotomy can be performed with the same - or even better - efficiency and safety. Decreasing the mortality and morbidity rates of esophageal surgery remains one of the goals for surgeons. Avoiding the consequences of thoracotomy [17] in fragile patients might be the first step toward this goal.

1. Esophagectomy

1.1. Technique

The preparation and draping are done as for the usual open procedure. The double-lumen tracheal tube has to be placed in perfect position. If not, incomplete lung collapse will result, making exposure of the mediastinum quite difficult. Unless the esophageal stricture is too tight, a NG-tube is introduced to help grasp the esophagus. The patient is in the left lateral position, tilting a little bit forward to facilitate exposure of the posterior mediastinum. The right arm must be elevated in order to leave the axilla free for possible insertion of additional trocar tubes. The operating table's bridge is adjusted in the appropriate position for possible thoracotomy, but is not elevated. The telescope is introduced into the 7th intercostal space (ICS) in the mid axillary line (AL). Two lung retractors are introduced in the anterior AL, usually in the 4th and 6th ICS. At least one 10 mm and one 5 mm retractor are required. However, the use of two 10 mm retractors is more effi-cient. They are held by an assistant or may be self-retaining. Time must be taken for correct exposure of the mediastinum. Gentle flattening of the lung with the retractor while the anesthesiologist aspirates the right bronchus helps keep the lung deflated. The esophageal dissection must be started only if a clear view of the mediastinum has been obtained. In cases of oozing or hemorrhage, hemostasis will be very difficult to achie-ve if vision is hindered by the lung. Usually, after a cer-tain amount of time, the lung remains retracted by itself, sometimes without need for retractors. Once exposure of the posterior mediastinum is correct, i.e when the esophagus can be clearly identified, 2 addi-tional 10 mm ports are introduced, one in the 5th ICS in the posterior AL, or even more posteriorly, and one in the 6th in the anterior AL for dissecting instruments and a clip-applier (Fig. 106). Even if one of the retrac-tors is a 5 mm one, it is more convenient to use only 10 mm trocar tubes, giving the surgeon the choice to change the position of the instruments or the telescope during the procedure. A grasping forceps is introduced through the posterior trocar tube. The mediastinal pleu-ra is grasped, pulled upward and opened with scissors. The pleural incision is continued from bottom to top, with or without cautery, depending on the degree of mediastinal inflammation. The lateral sides of the eso-phagus are loosened using blunt tip scissors or a dis-sector. Once partly freed, the esophagus is grasped with an esophageal forceps and pulled upward and backward. The forceps can be shifted along the length of the esophagus and is thus more convenient than a loop passed around the esophageal body which cannot be moved so easily. The hemostasis of esophageal ves-sels is achieved with cautery (Fig. 107) and clips (Fig. 108). The use of curved scissors and curved for-ceps is very helpful for dissection of the mediastinal side of the esophagus. This stage of the procedure is

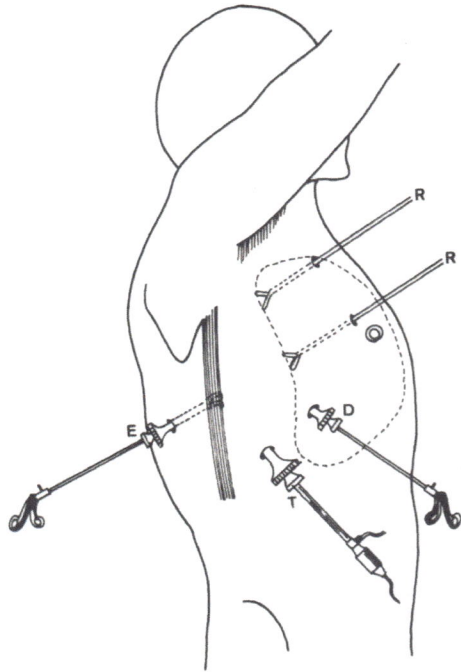

106

Fig. 106. Schematic illustration of trocar location. *T*: telescope, *D*: dissecting instruments, *E*: esophageal forceps, *R*: retractors

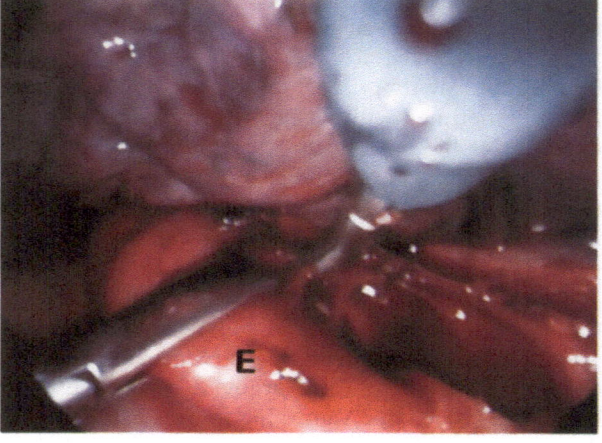

107

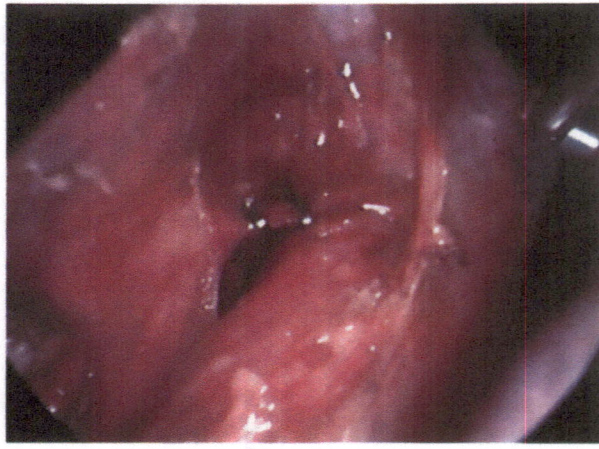

108

Fig. 107. Hemostasis of esophageal vessels using electocautery (*E* = Esophagus)

Fig. 108. Hemostasis of esophageal vessels using clips

sometimes made difficult by minor persistent oozing which requires frequent suction. In order to avoid an awkward inflation of the lung during suction, short aspiration periods must be used. Keeping one or two trocar tubes empty is also an efficient solution, allowing one to keep a permanent suction device in place. Once the esophagus has been mobilized up to its upper third, the azygos vein must be divided. Before doing

so, one has to be sure that the instruments will easily reach the upper part of the chest so they can be maneuvered safely, and that the vision is not too tangential as may occur in endomorphic patients. In this case, the 0° telescope must be changed for a 30° telescope, or must be introduced into the axilla, thus giving direct vision of the azygos. The blunt tip scissors are gently slipped under the mediastinal pleura which is divided up to the top of the chest (Fig. 109). The back of the vein is dissected using scissors and a dissector. Before engaging the endostapler, one has to be sure that the dissector tip is visible at the superior edge of the vein (Fig. 110) and that 2 cm of the azygos is totally dissected (Fig. 111). The vein is then divided using the vascular endostapler which must be introduced perpendicular to the vein, i.e through the port used for the telescope. Thus the telescope must be moved to another port and the previous 10 mm trocar of the telescope must be changed for a 12 mm one. In order to pass the stapler smoothly behind the azygos, the vein can be elevated with the dissector or with a loop. Once the vein is completely between the stapler's jaws, the stapler can be fired (Fig. 112). The division of the azygos vein allows one to end the dissection of the upper third of the esophagus (Fig. 112). Using the instrument locations described above, only the upper two-thirds of the esophagus can be dissected. For dissection of the lower third, the direction of the telescope and the instruments must be shifted 180°. For this stage, the operator should move to the patient's front, making maneuvering of the instruments easier. The esophageal dissection is continued downward to the diaphragme. The dissection of the lower third can be left incomplete if the esophagoplasty stage is conducted through a laparotomy, because the lower part of the esophagus is easy to mobilise via laparotomy. However, if esophagoplasty is conducted laparoscopically, it is easier to dissect the esophagus as far as possible via thoracoscopy. Once the esophagus is totally free, the esophagectomy can be ended through the cervicotomy or through the abdomen. A chest tube is put in place in the esophageal bed (Fig. 113).

The esophageal reconstruction is made using either colon or stomach according to the operator's choice and to the possibilities. A gastroplasty can be performed via laparoscopy, as described by Dallemagne et al [9]. However, this technique is time consuming and of no proven benefit, compared with the open technique.

1.2. Discussion

Until recently, there were only two ways to perform an esophagectomy, either through thoracotomy or without thoracotomy (EWT) using blunt dissection. The respiratory morbidity of open esophagectomy is high, ranging from 6% to 10% [29]. This high morbidity is partly responsible for the 6% to 15% mortality rate. Many techniques of EWT have been described since the initial report of Orringer [1, 30]. In some particular indications, such as caustic necrosis, blunt stripping can be easily performed without danger or risk of hemorrhage [15]. However, in most cases this blind technique does not allow sufficient control and the middle third of the esophagus remains hidden, even when using a large phrenotomy [12]. Although the blood vessels to the esophagus are small [28], there is considerable risk of hemorrhage. In Orringer's report, the average blood loss was 900 cc [31]. In a review of the literature, Liebermann-Meffert et al have noted a fatal hemorrage rate of 1.6% (most often due to injury of the azygos vein) and a tracheal tear rate of 3% [28]. Above all, the advantage in terms of respiratory morbidity has not been demonstrated. In a series of 304 EWT collected by Perrachai and Bardini, the pulmonary complications were as follows: tracheobronchial tear (1.5%), pleural effusion (17.8%), and operative mortality rate 10.3% [33]. Shahian et al have reported a respiratory morbidity rate higher (although not-significantly) after EWT than after open esophagectomy [37].

For 3 years, Buess et al have improved the technique of EWT by the use of an "endoscopic microsurgical dissection of the esophagus" through mediastinoscopy [6, 24]. The operating mediastinoscope is introduced into the posterior mediastinum through a left cervicotomy. It has a central working channel and its optic offers a 2 to 4 enlarged image, thus allowing accurate dissection of vessels and nerves. The esophagus is dissected downward and removed transhiatally through a laparotomy. After having shown this method to be efficient and safe in an animal model [24], Buess et al reported a serie of 17 cases with no operative mortality and with minimal blood loss (< 200 cc) [6].

The thoracoscopic approach for esophagectomy is another way of trying to reduce, if not solve, the problem of respiratory morbidity. The technique is too recent to form an opinion about the results. Compared with the mediastinoscopic approach, the thoracoscopic approach has the advantage of giving a wider view of the pleural cavity and of the mediastinum. Thus, it allows for a more extended excision than in mediastinoscopy . An evaluation of both techniques are necessary to decide whether these methods are complementary or opposed.

2. Truncal vagotomy

2.1. Technique

Although it is usual to approach the vagus nerves through the left thorax [27], it is often more convenient to perform the vagotomy through a right thoracoscopy [16]. This is because, though the lower esophagus and vagus nerves are sometimes clearly

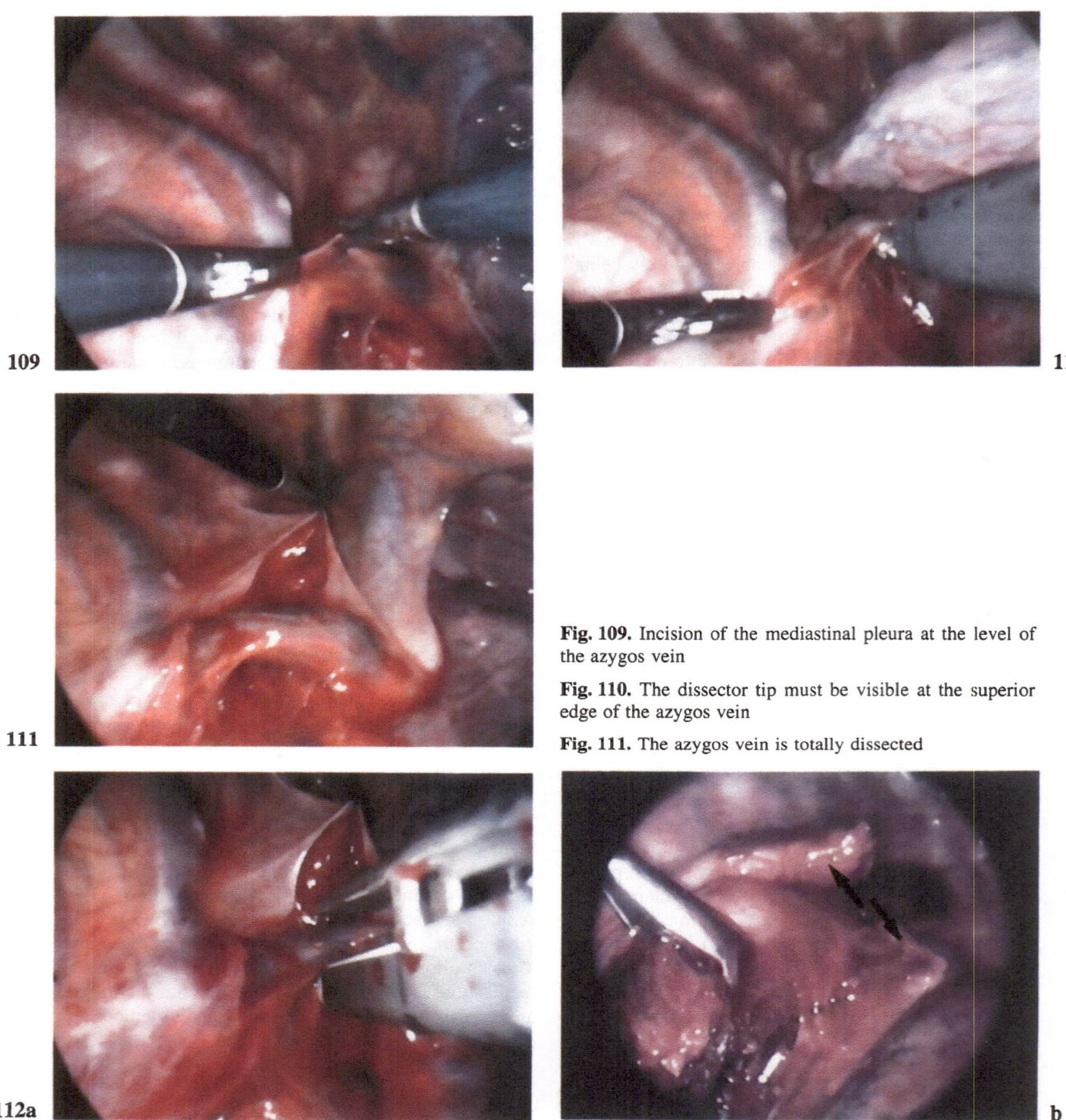

109

11

111

112a

b

Fig. 109. Incision of the mediastinal pleura at the level of the azygos vein

Fig. 110. The dissector tip must be visible at the superior edge of the azygos vein

Fig. 111. The azygos vein is totally dissected

Fig. 112. a The endostapler can be applied, **b** View of the divided vein *(arrows)*

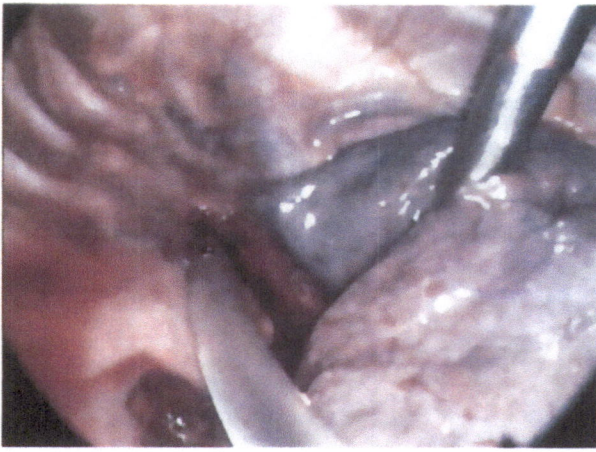

Fig. 113. Chest tube in the esophageal bed

visible through a left thoracoscopic approach, it is usually necessary to free the inferior pulmonary ligament.

However, even after freeing this ligament, identification of the esophagus can be difficult when it is hidden by an enlarged aorta in an old patient or because of particular anatomic conditions, e.g a scoliosis. On the other hand, the right thoracoscopic approach always makes it possible to identify the vagus nerves. One only has to be sure to perform the vagotomy as low as possible to avoid dividing not only a branch of the esophageal plexus but the whole vagal trunk [40].

The patient is in the left lateral position, with his arm hanging down or elevated, depending on the operator's preference. Double-lumen tracheal intubation is essential to good exposure of the posterior mediastinum. Usually, 4 trocar tubes are required: one 10 mm port in the 5th ICS in the mid AL for the telescope, one 10 mm in the 5th ICS in the anterior AL for a lung retractor, one 5 mm in the 6th ICS in the posterior AL for a grasping forceps and another 5 mm in the 6th ICS for dissecting instruments and scissors. The mediastinal pleura is opened at the level of the lower esophagus (Fig. 114). The right trunk is generally immediately visible on the right side of the esophagus (Fig. 115). The left vagus nerve is usually more distal. In some cases, it is necessary to introduce an esophageal grasping forceps to pull the esophagus backward to expose the nerve. Once the two trunks have been identified, they must be dissected for a 4-5 cm length downward, thus making sure that no branch is ignored. Then, they are clipped and divided (Fig. 116). The procedure is usually bloodless. A single small size chest tube is sufficient.

2.2. Discussion

The endoscopic approach to the vagus nerves is not new as the procedure has been performed through the laparoscope [23] and more recently through the thoracoscope [8]. Truncal vagotomy is the most efficient vagotomy. Parietal cell vagotomies have a low morbidity rate, but are known to have a recurrence rate of 15% to 28% after 10 years [18]. However, the adverse effects of truncal vagotomy make its routine use questionable. Diarrhea may occur in 5% to 9% of patients, severe in 2% [18]. Troubles in gastric emptying occur in about 10% of patients if a pyloromyotomy does not complete the procedure [10, 19]. Theoretically, methods exist to solve the problem of gastric emptying after a thoracic vagotomy. The pylorus can be dilated endoscopically using balloon catheters [36]. Although Kozarek has reported a 76% technical success rate in pyloric stenosis, the objective relief at 3 months was only 37% [25]. Another minimally invasive technique would be to perform a laparoscopic pyloromyotomy, as recently proposed by Alain et al [2]. However, this method is not suitable for patients with previous abdominal operations.

For all these reasons, it would seem to be wrong to consider this operation as the standard approach for vagotomy simply because it is an easy and appealing method. However, thoracoscopy is the ideal approach in patients for whom a thoracic vagotomy remains indicated, i.e patients with recurrent peptic ulcer with previous abdominal surgery. It is also the method of choice for vagotomy used to complement of total duodenal diversion [34]. Although no data is available with regard to the morbidity rate, it should be less than that in thoracotomy. In a report of 47 patients who were operated via left thoracotomy, Lehr et al noted 15 cases of pleural effusion and 5 cases of atelectasis, with a mean hospital stay of 11 days [27].

3. Other procedures

3.1. Benign tumors of the esophagus

3.1.1. Technique

The preparation and first stages are as for thoracoscopic esophagectomy. The approach is a right thoracoscopy, with double-lumen intubation and an NG-tube into the esophagus. The procedure is quite easy in the case of a small tumor located on the right side of the esophagus. It can be more problematic if the tumor is large or located on the left side (Fig. 117).

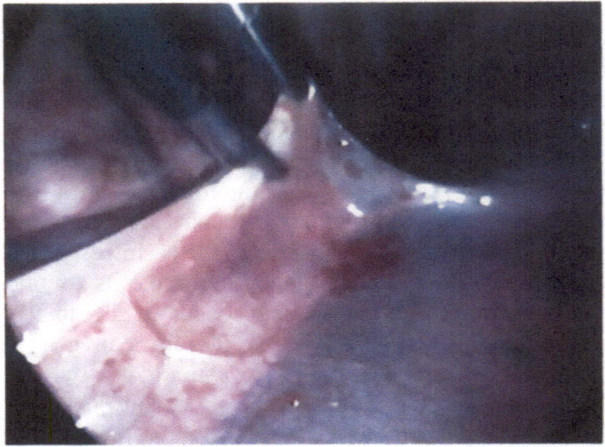

114

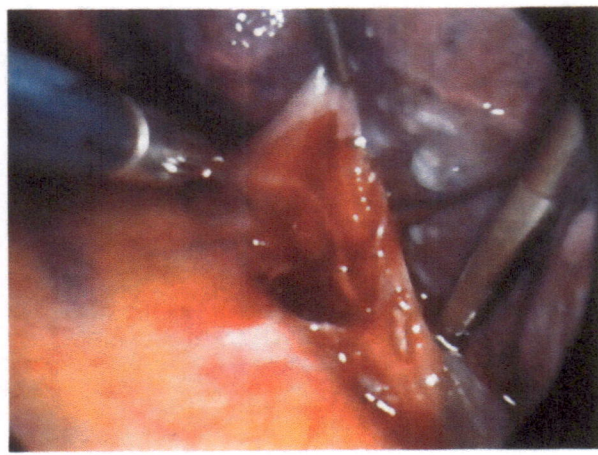

11

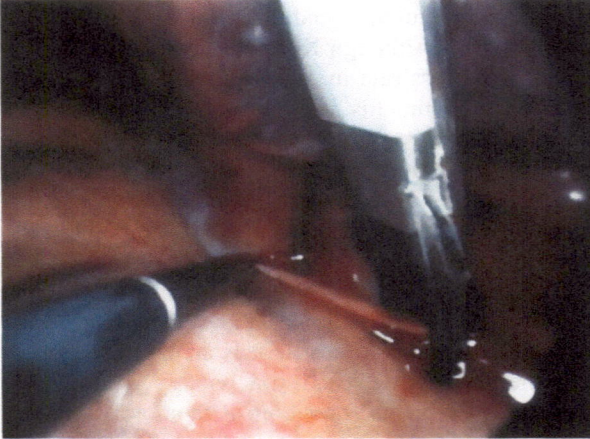

116

Fig. 114. Right thoracoscopic approach for vagotomy. Opening of the mediastinal pleura

Fig. 115. Right thoracoscopic view of the esophagus and the right vagus nerve

Fig. 116. Dissection of the left vagus trunk through right thoracoscopy

In this case, the esophagus must be almost completely mobilized lengthwise in order to be rotated, thus exposing the tumor on the right side of the mediastinum.

One problem is that the tumor is usually not clearly visible on the esophageal wall, and that the operator is not helped by manual palpation. It may be helpful to perform a perioperative esophageal endoscopy in order to precisely locate the limits of the tumor. These limits are then marked off on the esophageal wall using electrocautery. The muscular layer is then opened with blunt tip scissors, their direction being perpendicular to the esophageal wall. Once the tumor appears between the muscular fibers, it is caught with a grasping forceps or a wire is passed through it using a straight needle (Fig. 118). The tumor is pulled upward and the dissection is continued using the same principles as in open surgery (Fig. 119). Compared with open chest surge-

ry, the main problem is not to lacerate the fibers, since the esophagus cannot be firmly held as in conventional surgery and tends to slide and twist under the scissor-tips. Laceration of the muscular fibers may result in a difficult repair, if the verges of the tumor excision are not clean. Once the tumor has been removed, one can check to see if the mucosa has been opened or not, by injecting methyl-blue through the NG-tube. However this test, if positive, will make repair of the mucosal wound difficult by giving a blue coloration to the whole operating field. It seems more convenient to inject gas through the endoscope and ask the endoscopist to look carefully at the mucosa. Then, the muscular layer is closed with a continuous suture (Fig. 120) using the technique described on page 13. At the end of the procedure, the tumor is removed through a short counterincision in the axilla. A chest tube is placed in the posterior mediastinum.

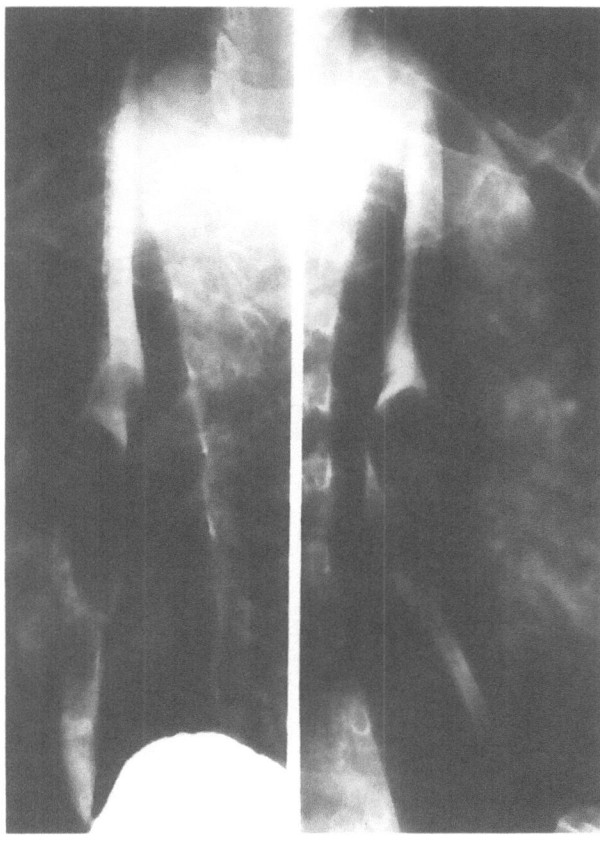

Fig. 117. Large esophageal leiomyoma located on the left side, removed through right thoracoscopic approach

3.1.2. Discussion

Benign tumors of the esophagus, i.e mainly leiomyomas and cysts, are rare. They seldom give rise to symptoms (about one third of the patients [3]) and thus their surgical treatment may seem out of proportion to their benign nature [14]. However, complications such as an increase in size, causing obstruction and pulmonary disorders or even malignant forms, have been reported [3]. Unless contraindicated, these tumors are therefore usually removed. Generally, a small lateral thoracotomy does not allow sufficient control of the esophagus, in which case a large thoracotomy is performed. The thoracoscopic approach is well suited to the benign nature of these tumors.

3.2. Miscellaneous

Although thoracoscopic treatment of esophageal diseases is quite new, one can assume that numerous applications will soon appear. Presently, these applications have only been suggested or outlined in case reports.

3.2.1. Treatment of esophageal perforation

Esophageal perforations are often recognized late, especially spontaneous perforations (Boerhaave's syndrome). Because of their extreme seriousness, with a mortality rate ranging between 20 and 30%, agressive treatment is most often the only choice, i.e removal of all infected and necrotic tissues, closure and drainage of the perforation and sometimes esophageal exclusion [13]. This is better achieved through thoracotomy. When the diagnosis is made within 24-48 hours, various treatments can been proposed: either conservative management by pleural drainage alone, or aggressive management with thoracotomy for debridement and an attempt to repair the esophagus. In these cases of early diagnosed perforations, the thoracoscopic approach can be useful. It allows one to aspirate the pleural effusion, suture the perforation or put a T-tube into it as well as place an irrigation system [20].

3.2.2. Treatment of esophageal motor disorders

Laparoscopic myotomy is now a common procedure for achalasia [37]. Theoretically, a myotomy is also feasable through the thoracoscope [16]. However it is probably not the best approach, since it is generally agreed that a myotomy for achalasia should be combined with an antireflux procedure [5]. Furthermore, most surgeons consider that the distal extent of the myotomy should carried into the stomach for at least 1 to 2 cm to avoid the risk of leaving the esophageal obstruction unrelieved. Perrachia et al have recently reported a 47% rate of incomplete distal myotomy in patients treated for recurrent symptoms after esophagomyotomy [32]. Performing a perfect myotomy thoracoscopically would require wide opening of the diaphragm in order to expose the esophagogastric junction and the stomach. This has been demonstrated as possible in animal models [26], but is not recommended as a routine. However, in patients with previous abdominal surgery, this alternative should be considered. The thoracoscopic approach may also be indicated for very rare cases of high-amplitude peristaltic esophageal contractions (nutcracker esophagus) in which an extensive esophagomyotomy has proved to be effective [39, 43].

3.3.3. Other indications

Various procedures have been reported: excision of esophageal diverticula, treatment of postoperative

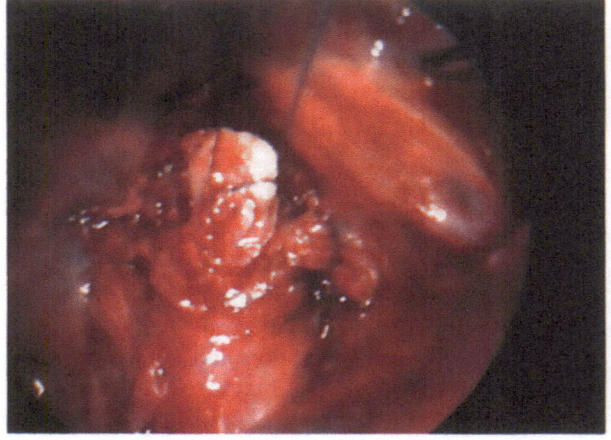

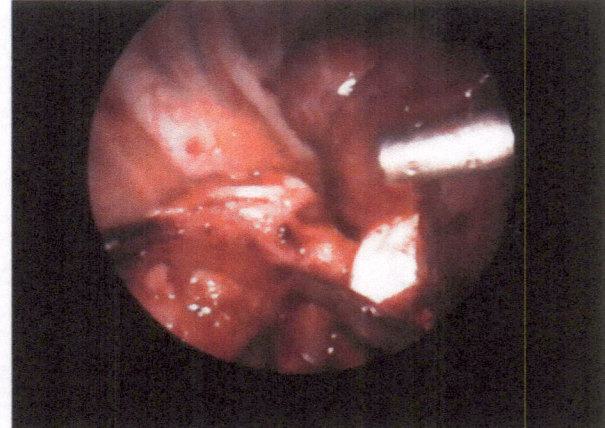

118

119

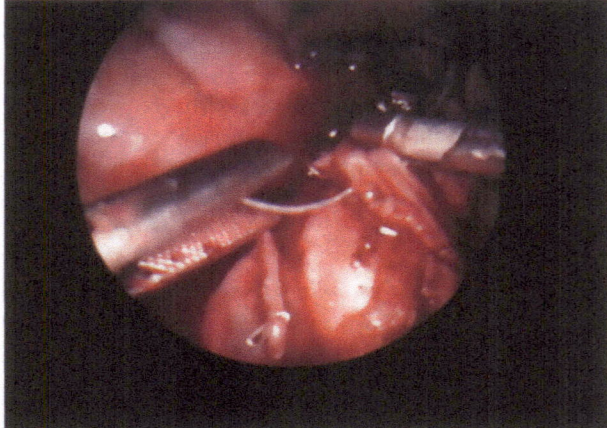

120

Fig. 118. Removal of a small leimyoma of the esophagus. A wire is passed through it for better exposure

Fig. 119. Removal of a large leiomyoma of the esophagus. The integrity of the mucosa is checked with lighting through the esophagoscope

Fig. 120. Closure of the esophageal wall

chylothorax [21] etc. Laparoscopic repair of diaphragmatic hernia has been reported [7]. In some cases, the thoracoscopic approach might be indicated, but further experimental works and evaluation are required in these fields.

4. Prospects in endoscopic esophageal surgery

Endoscopic surgery of the esophagus is in it's initial stages. Articles on clinical cases are being published now that it has been shown to be feasible in animals [6, 8, 9]. It is too early to have an opinion concerning the benefits in terms of morbidity and survival. However, in regard to morbidity, the benefit seems obvious. Avoiding the consequences of thoracotomy in fragile patients is already an advance. Nevertheless, some questions will need to be answered in the near future:

1) What are the respective indications for the mediastinoscopic and thoracoscopic approaches?

The mediastinoscopic technique has been demonstrated to be safe, especially with regard to the control of perioperative hemorrage [6]. There is no need for selective tracheal intubation, thus decreasing the risk of atelectasis. However, it does not allow a view of the surrounding mediastinal structures, thus making carcinologic surgery almost impossible. Buess et al justify their approach by the fact that the surgical resection of esophageal cancer is primarily palliative [6]. This opinion is supported by others [4], but some surgeons have shown a significant benefit in en-bloc esophagectomy for early stage (N0 and N1) carcinomas [41]. Although extensive node dissection has been shown to be feasible through thoracoscopy in animal models [16], it is not known whether such dissection can be safely performed on patients.

2) Is there a place for thoracoscopy in preoperative staging?

As far as lymph-node involvement is concerned, no ideal pre-operative investigation has been found. Endosonography has a better accuracy than computed tomography [15]. Tio et al have demonstrated that endoscopic ultrasonography can detect periesophageal nodes in most cases (95%). Nevertheless, the specificity is poor: 50% of the nodes are in fact only inflammatory [42]. Tio et al have suggested performing sonographically guided biopsies to enhance the accuracy of endosonography. Thoracoscopic node picking (Fig. 121) might give the best results (laparoscopic staging has already been shown to be very effective in cancer of the cardia [44]) but the procedure is probably more invasive than endosonography. However, in some cases where the tumoral stricture is too tight to allow passage of the sonographic probe, or in case of doubt, thoracoscopy may be indicated.

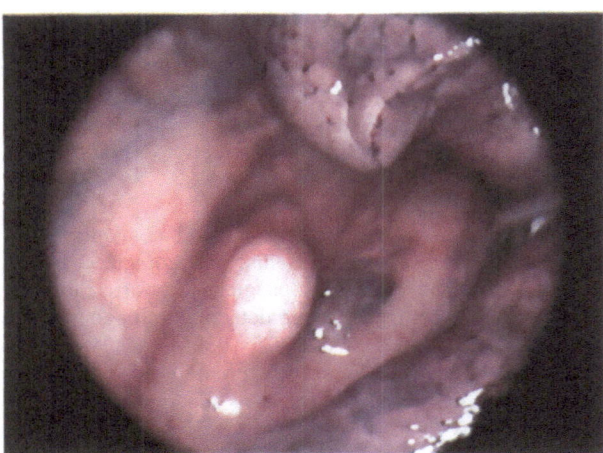

Fig. 121. View of a large paraesophageal node

References

1. Akiyama H, Tsurumaru M, Ono Y, Udagawa H, Matsuda M, Kajiyama Y (1991) Transoral esophagectomy. Surg Gyn Obstet 173 : 399-400
2. Alain JL, Grousseau D, Terrier G (1991) Extramucosal pylorotomy by laparoscopy. Surg Endosc 5 : 174-175
3. Arnorsson T, Aberg C, Aberg T (1984) Benign tumors of the esophagus and esophageal cysts. Scand J Thorac Cardiovasc Surg 18 : 145-150
4. Barbier PA, Becker CD, Wagner HE (1988) Esophageal carcinoma: patient selection for transhiatal esophagectomy. A prospective analysis of 50 consecutive cases. World J Surg 12 : 263-269
5. Bonavina L, Nosadini A, Bardini R, Baessato M, Peracchia A (1992) Primary treatment of esophageal achalasia. Long-term results of myotomy and Dor fundoplication. Arch Surg 127 : 222-227
6. Buess GF, Becker HD, Naruhn MB, Mentges BR (1991) Endoscopic esophagectomy without thoracotomy. Problems in General Surgery 8 : 478-486
7. Campos LI, Sipes EK (1991) Laparoscopic repair of diaphragmatic hernia. J Laparoendosc Surg 1: 369-373
8. Chisholm EM, Chung SCS, Sunderland GT, Leong HT, Li AKC (1992) Thoracoscopic vagotomy: a new use for the laparoscope. Br J Surg 79 : 254
9. Dallemagne B, Weerts JM, Jehaes G, Markiewicz S, Bona S (1992) Subtotal esophagectomy by thoracoscopy and laparoscopy. Minimal Invasive Therapy 1 :183-185
10. Dragstedt LR, Lulu DJ (1974) Truncal vagotomy and pyloroplasty: critical evaluation of one hundred cases. Ann Surg 128 : 344-346
11. Geagea T (1991) Laparoscopic Nissen's fundoplication: preliminary report on ten cases. Surg Endosc 5 : 170-173
12. Goldberg M, Freeman J, Gullane PJ, Patterson A, Todd TRJ, McShane D (1989) Transhiatal esophagectomy with gastric transposition for pharyngeal malignant disease. J Thorac Cardiovasc Surg 97 : 327-333
13. Gossot D, Sarfati E, Celerier M (1986) Les perforations de l'oesophage thoracique. A propos de 14 cas opérés. J Chir 123 : 607-610
14. Gossot D, Sarfati E, Celerier M (1987) Faut-il opérer les tumeurs bénignes de l'oesophage? Med Chir Dig 16 : 483-484
15. Gossot D, Sarfati E, Celerier M (1987) Early blunt esophagectomy in severe caustic burns of the upper digestive tract. Report of 29 cases. J Thorac Cardiovasc Surg 94 : 188-191
16. Gossot D, Ghnassia MD, Debiolles H, Chourrout Y, Bonnichon JM, Sarfati E, Celerier M, Revillon Y (1992) Thoracoscopic dissection of the esophagus: an experimental study. Surg Endosc 6 : 59-61
17. Hallfeldt KKJ, Knoeffel WTK, Thetter O, Deubler E, Schweiberer L (1990) Respiratory function after thoracic operations. Ann Thorac Surg 50 : 684-688
18. Hoffmann J, Jensen HE, Christiansen J, Olesen A, Loud FB, Hauch O (1989) Prospective controlled vagotomy trial for duodenal ulcer. Results after 11-15 years. Ann Surg 20 : 40-45
19. Howlett PJ, Shewer MJ, Barber DC, Ward AS, Perez Avila CA, Duthie ML (1976) Gastric emptying in control subjects and patients with duodenal ulcer before and after vagotomy. Gut, 17 :542-550
20. Hutter JA, Fenn A, Brainbridge MV (1985) The management of spontaneous oesophageal perforation by thoracoscopy and irrigation. Br J Surg 72 : 208-209
21. Inderbitzi E, Krebs Th, Stirnemann P, Althaus U (1992) Treatment of postoperative chylothorax by fibrin glue application under thoracoscopic view using local anesthesia. J Thorac Cardiovasc Surg 104 : 209-210
22. Isono K, Onoda S, Ishikawa T, Sato H, Nakayama K (1982) Studies of the causes of death from esophageal carcinoma. Cancer 49 : 2173-2179

23. Katkhouda N, Mouiel J (1991) A new technique of surgical treatment of chronic duodenal ulcer without laparotomy by videocoelioscopy. Am J Surg 161 : 361-364

24. Kipfmüller K, Naruhn M, Melzer A, Kessler S, Buess G (1989) Endoscopic microsurgical dissection of the esophagus. Results in an animal model. Surg Endosc 3 : 63-69

25. Kozarek RA (1986) Hydrostatic balloon dilatation of gastrointestinal stenoses: a national survey. Gastrointestinal Endosc 32 : 15-19

26. Leahy PF, Pennino RP, Hinshaw Jr, O'Connor TP, Lanzafame RF (1990) Minimally invasive esophagogastrectomy: an approcah to esophagogastrectomy through the left thorax. J Laparoendosc Surg 1 : 59-62

27. Lehr L, Pichlmayr R (1982) Low risk thoracic vagotomy for anastomotic ulceration. World J Surg 6 : 93-97

28. Liebermann-Meffert DAI, Luescher URS, Neff UR, Ruedi TP, Allgoxer M (1987) Esophagectomy without thoracotomy: is there a risk of intramediastinal bleeding? Ann Surg 206 :184-192

29. Nishi M, Hiramatsu Y, Hioki K, Kojima Y, Sanadra T, Yamanaka H, Yamamoto M (1988) Risk factors in relation to postoperative complications in patients undergoing esophagectomy or gastrectomy for cancer. Ann Surg 207 : 148-154

30. Orringer MB, Sloan H (1978) Esophagectomy without thoracotomy. J Thorac Cardiovasc Surg 76 : 643-654

31. Orringer MB, Orringer JS (1983) Esophagectomy without thoracotomy: a dangerous operation? J Thorac Carfiovasc Surg 85 : 72-80

32. Peracchia A, Bonavina L, Nosadini A, Baessato M, Bardini R (1990) Management of recurent symptoms after esophagomyotomy for achalasia. Dis Esoph 3 : 25-28

33. Peracchia A, Bardini R (1986) Total esophagectomy without thoracotomy: results of a european questionnaire (GEEMO). Int Surg 71 : 171-175

34. Perniceni T, Gayet B, Fekete F (1988) Total duodenal diversion in the treatment of complicated peptic oesophagitis. Br J Surg 75 : 1108-1111

35. Pradhan GN, Eng JB, Sabanathan S (1989) Left thoracotomy approach for resection of carcinoma of the esophagus. Surg Gyn Obstet 168 : 49-53

36. Schmüdderich W, Harloff M, Riemann JF (1989) Through-the-scope balloon dilatation of benign pyloric stenoses. Endoscopy 21 : 7-10

37. Shahian DM, Neptune WB, Ellis FH, Watkins E (1986) Transthoracic versus extrathoracic esophagectomy: mortality, morbidity and long-term survival. Ann Thorac Surg 41 : 237-246

38. Shimi S, Nathanson LK, Cushieri A (1991) Laparoscopic cardiomyotomy for achalasia. J R Coll Surg Edinb 36 : 152-154

39. Shimi S, Nathanson LK, Cushieri A (1992) Thoracoscopic long œsophageal myotomy for nuteracker œsophagus : initial experience of a new surgical approach. Br J Surg 79 : 533-536

40. Skandalakis LJ, Gray SW, Skandalakis JE (1986) The history and surgical anatomy of the vagus nerves. Surg Gyn Obstet 162 : 75-85

41. Skinner DB, Ferguson MK, Soriano A, Little AG, Staszak VM (1986) Selection of operation for esophageal cancer based on staging. Ann Surg 204 : 391-400

42. Tio TL, Coene PPL, Luiken GJ, Tytgat GN (1990) Endosonography in the clinical staging of oesophagogastric carcinoma. Gastrointestinal Endosc 36 : 2-10

43. Traube M, Tummala V, Baue A, McCallum AW (1987) Surgical myotomy in patients with high-amplitude peristaltic esophageal contractions. Manometric and clinical effects. Digestive Disease and Sciences 32 : 16-21

44. Watt I, Stewart I, Anderson D, Bell G, Anderson J (1989) Laparoscopy, ultrasound and computed tomography in cancer of the esophagus and gastric cardia: a prospective comparison for detecting intra-abdominal metastases. Br J Surg 76 : 1036-1039

45. Ziegler K, Sanft C, Semsch B, Friedrich M, Gregor M, Riechken EO: Endosonography is superior to computed tomography in staging tumors of the esophagus and the cardia (1988). Gastroenterology 94 : A 51-57 (Abstr)

Index

THORACOSCOPY

Thoracoscopy is a valuable method for chest surgery offering various advantages like fewer operative complications and quick recovery time. The OLYMPUS Thoracoscopy System features both 100 % distortion-free hard optic technology and unsurpassed fiberoptics. The deflectable Thoracofiberscope allows full access to all areas which are hard to reach and minimizes the number of punctures required.

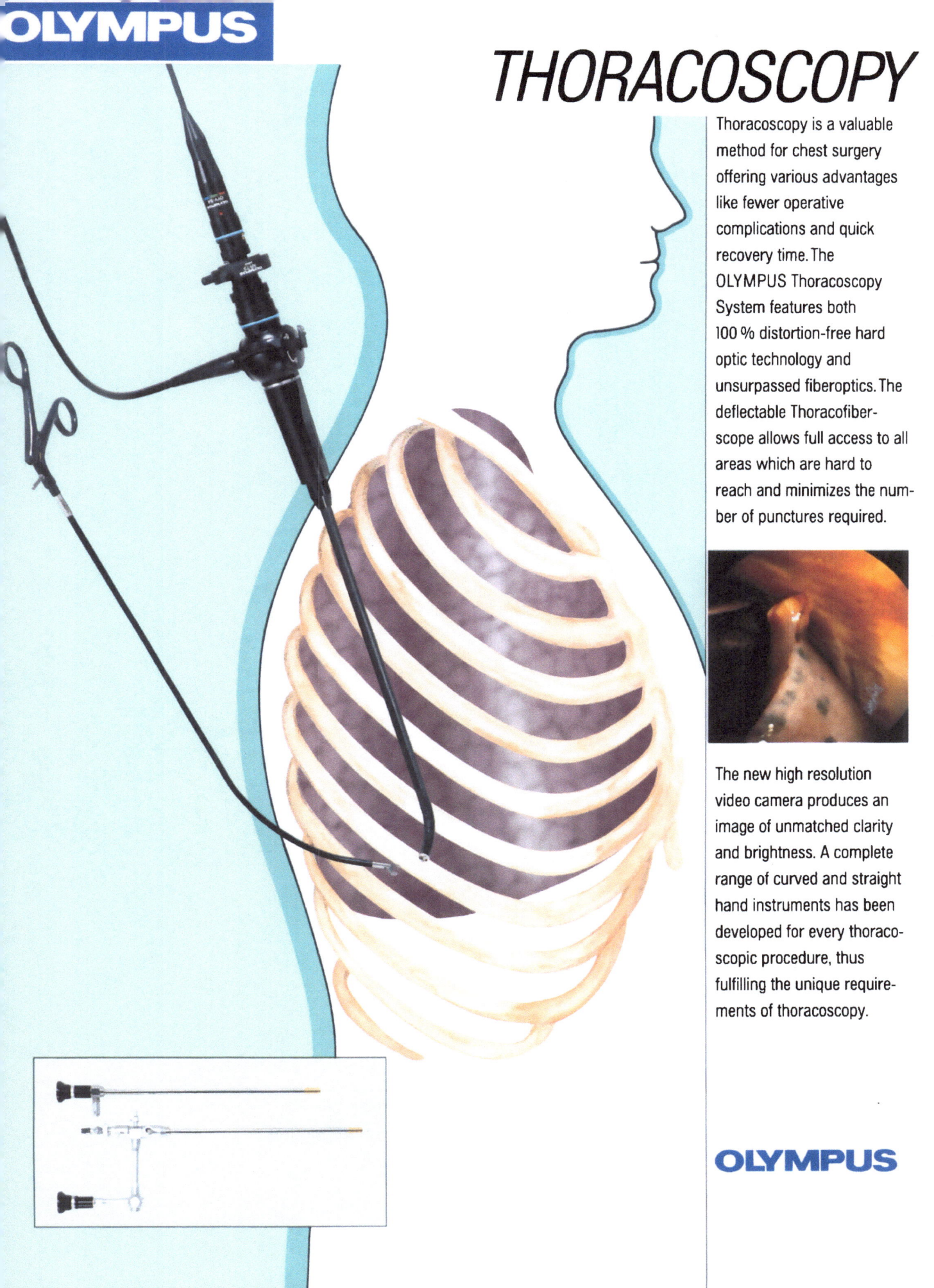

The new high resolution video camera produces an image of unmatched clarity and brightness. A complete range of curved and straight hand instruments has been developed for every thoracoscopic procedure, thus fulfilling the unique requirements of thoracoscopy.

Achevé d'imprimer par   Corlet, Imprimeur, S.A.
14110 Condé-sur-Noireau (France)
N° d'Éditeur : 617 - N° d'Imprimeur : 6199 - Dépôt légal : décembre 1992

Imprimé en C.E.E.